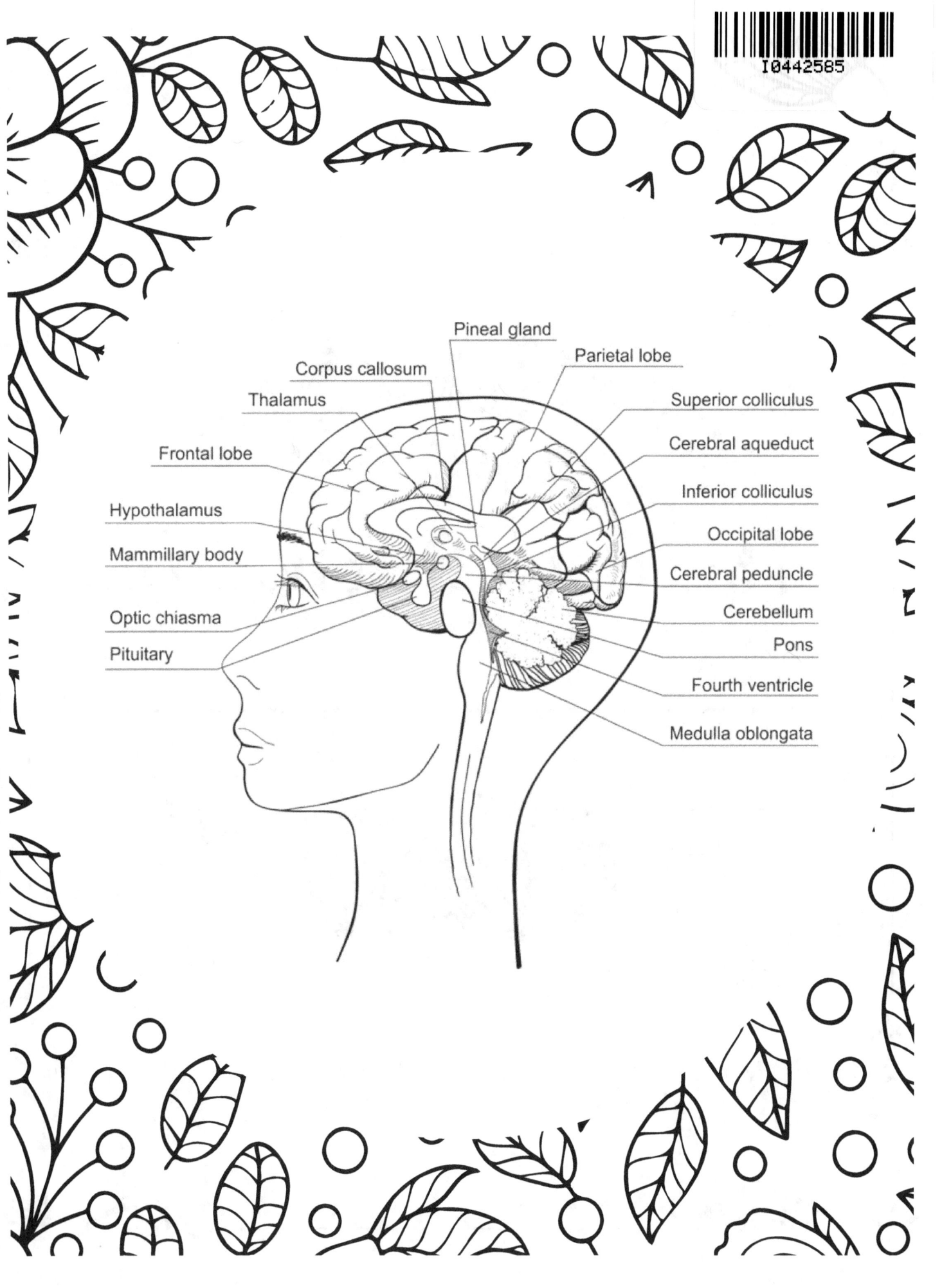

This Book Belongs To

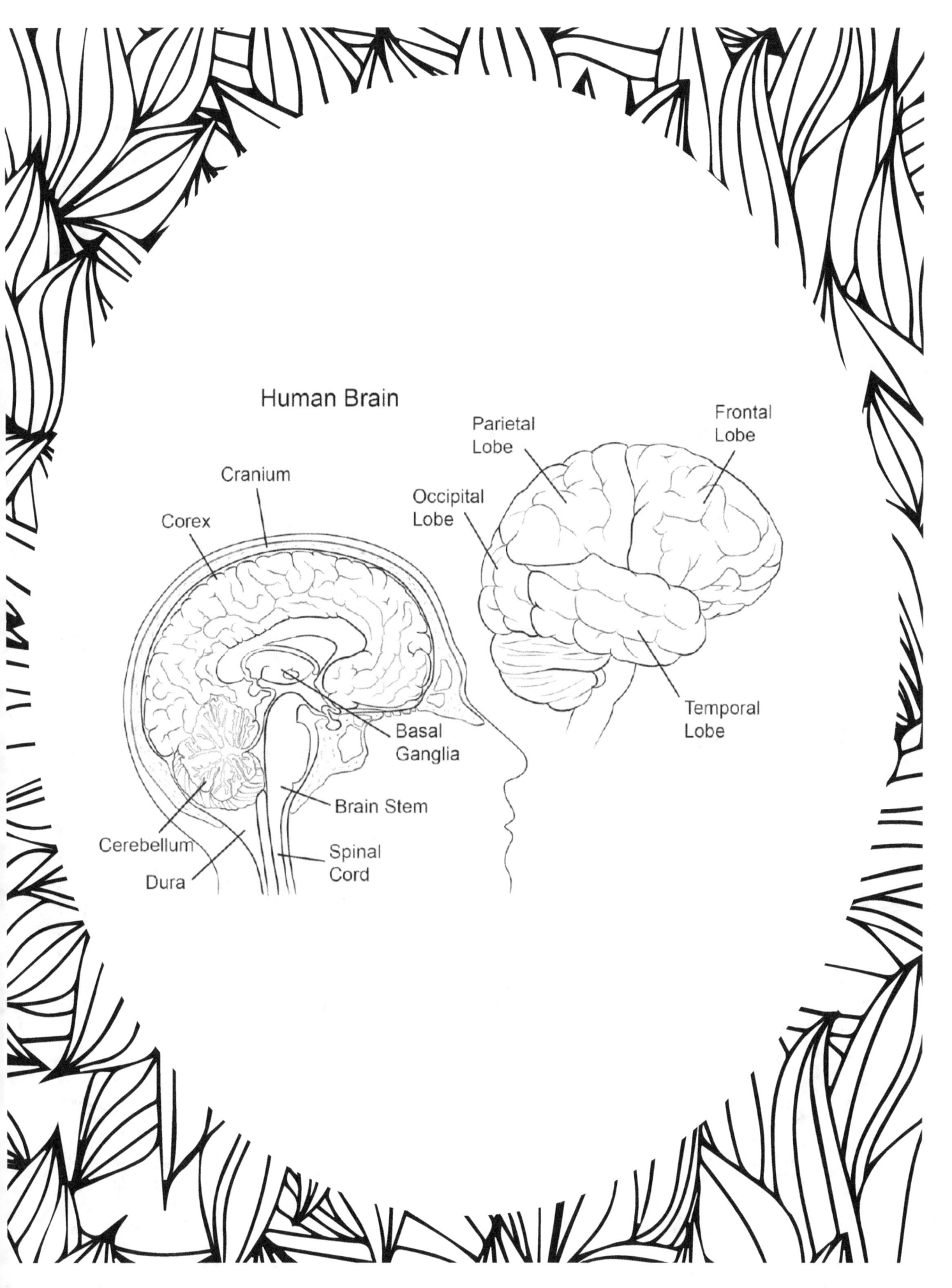

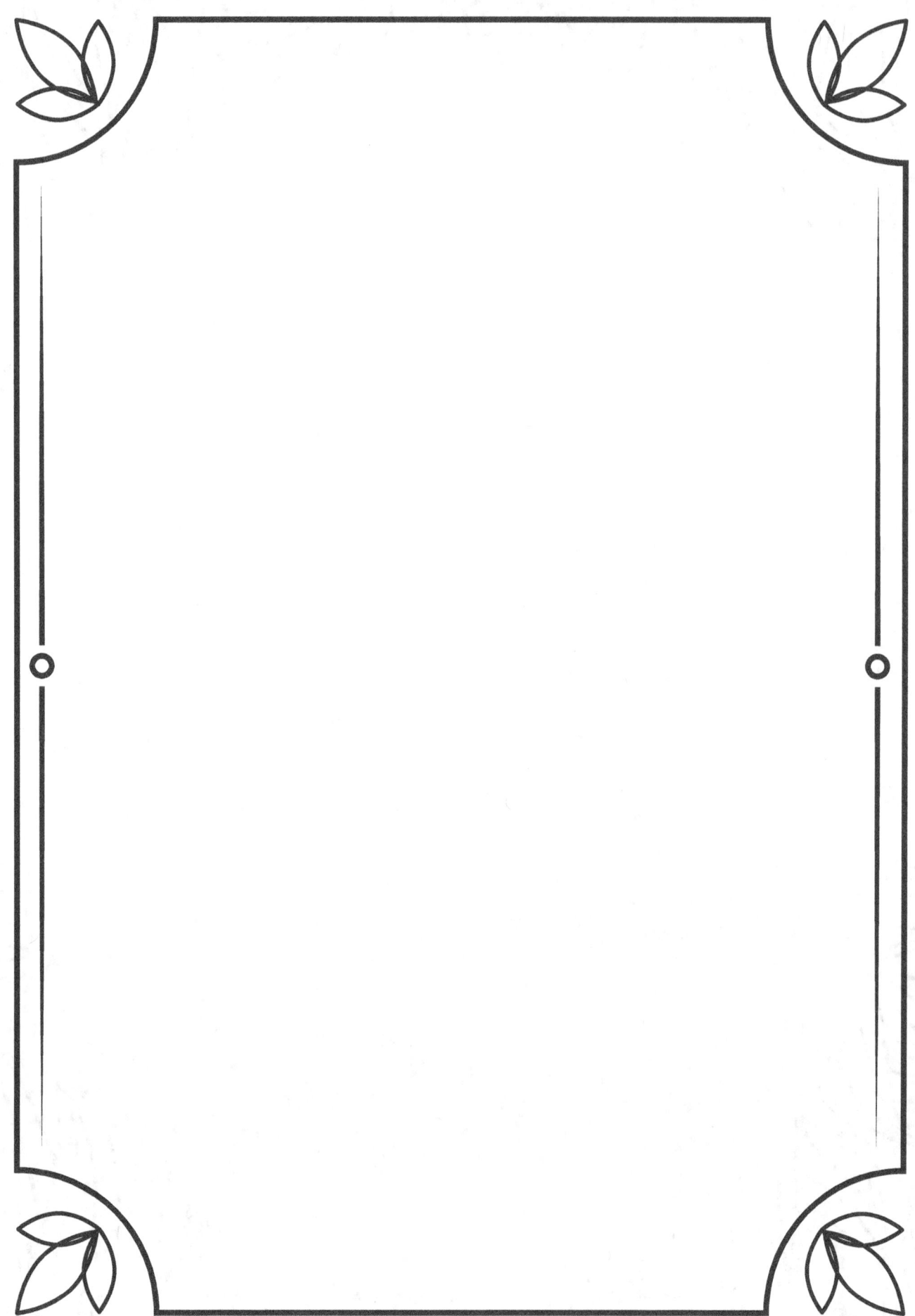

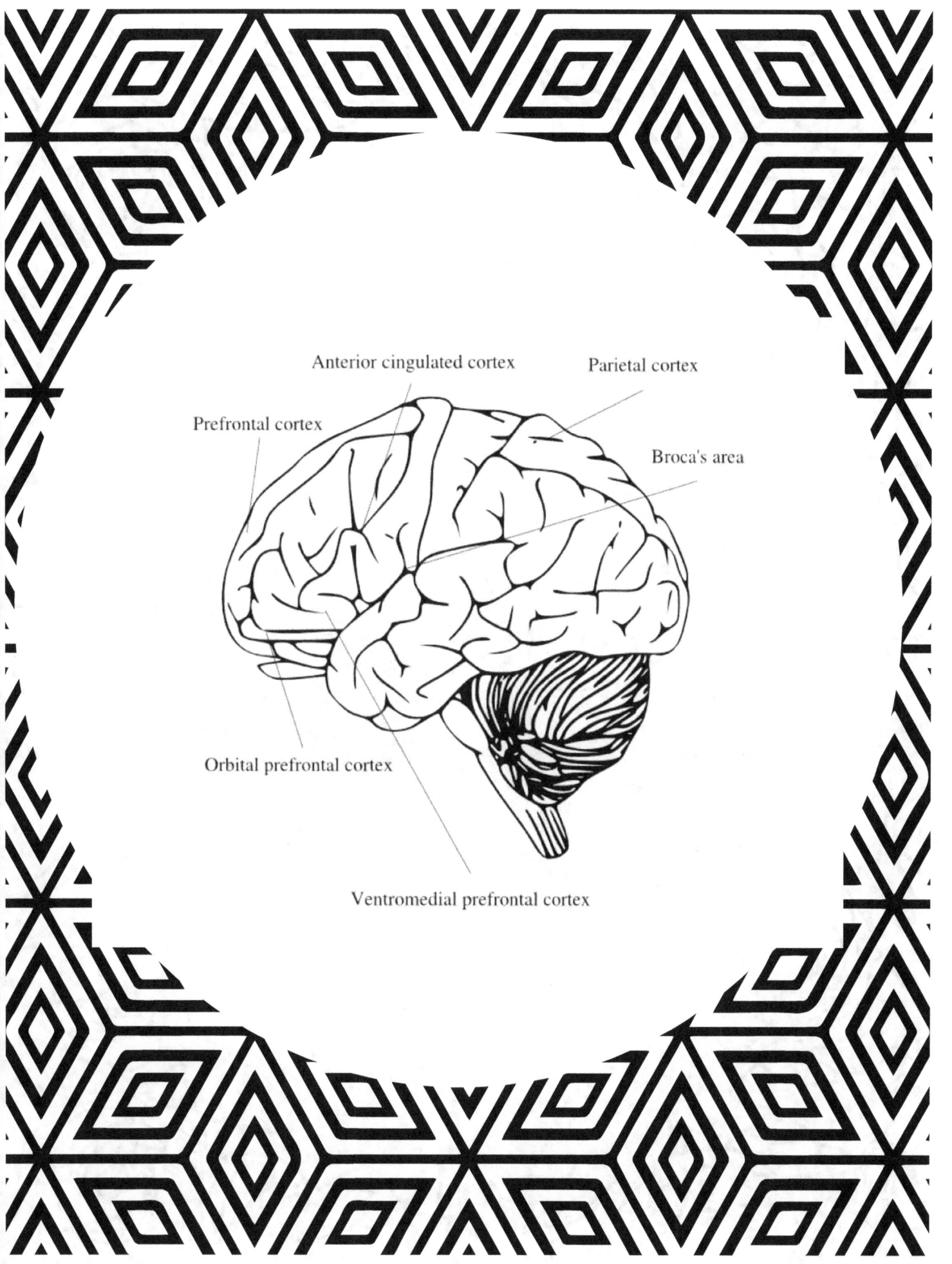

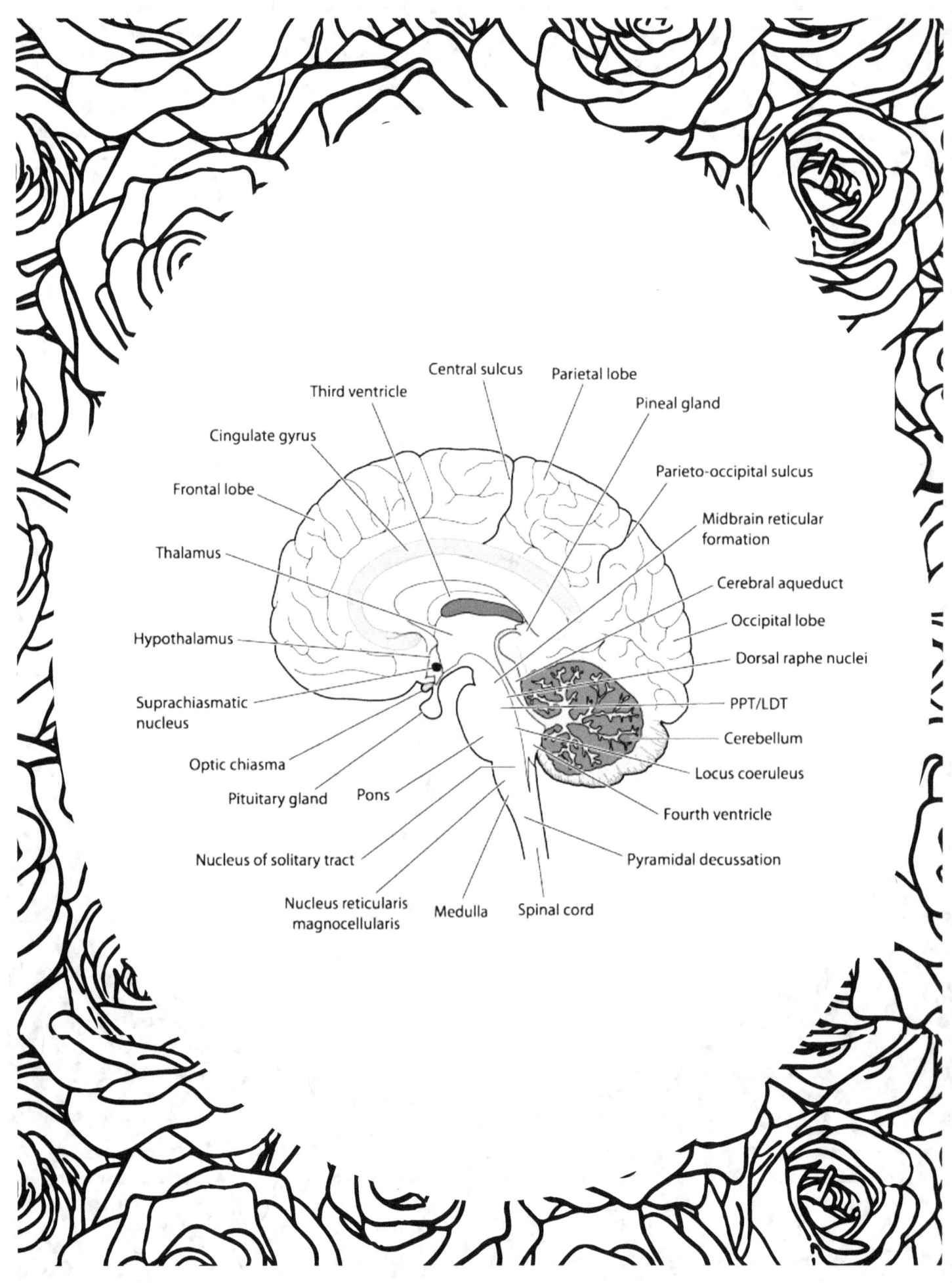

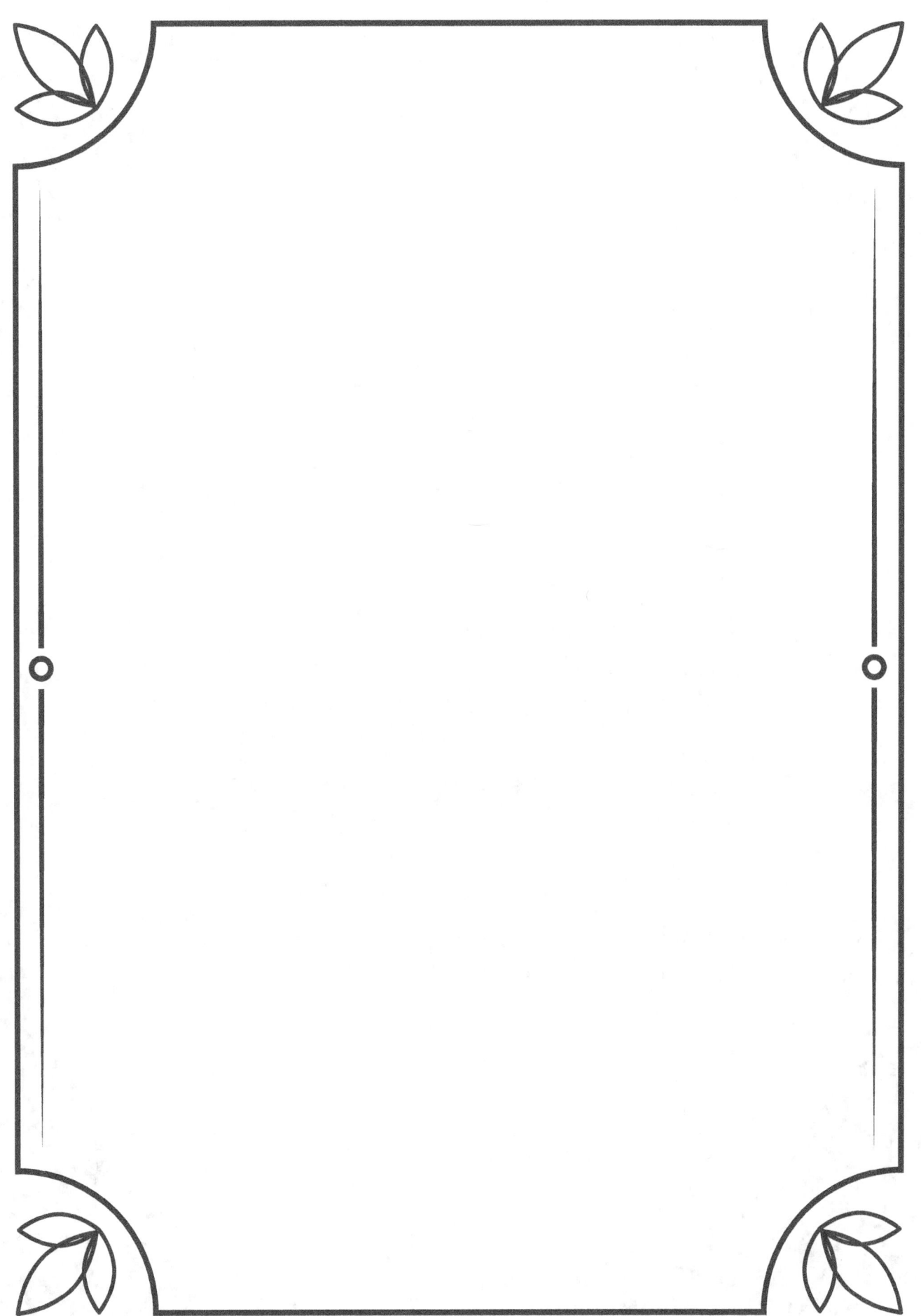

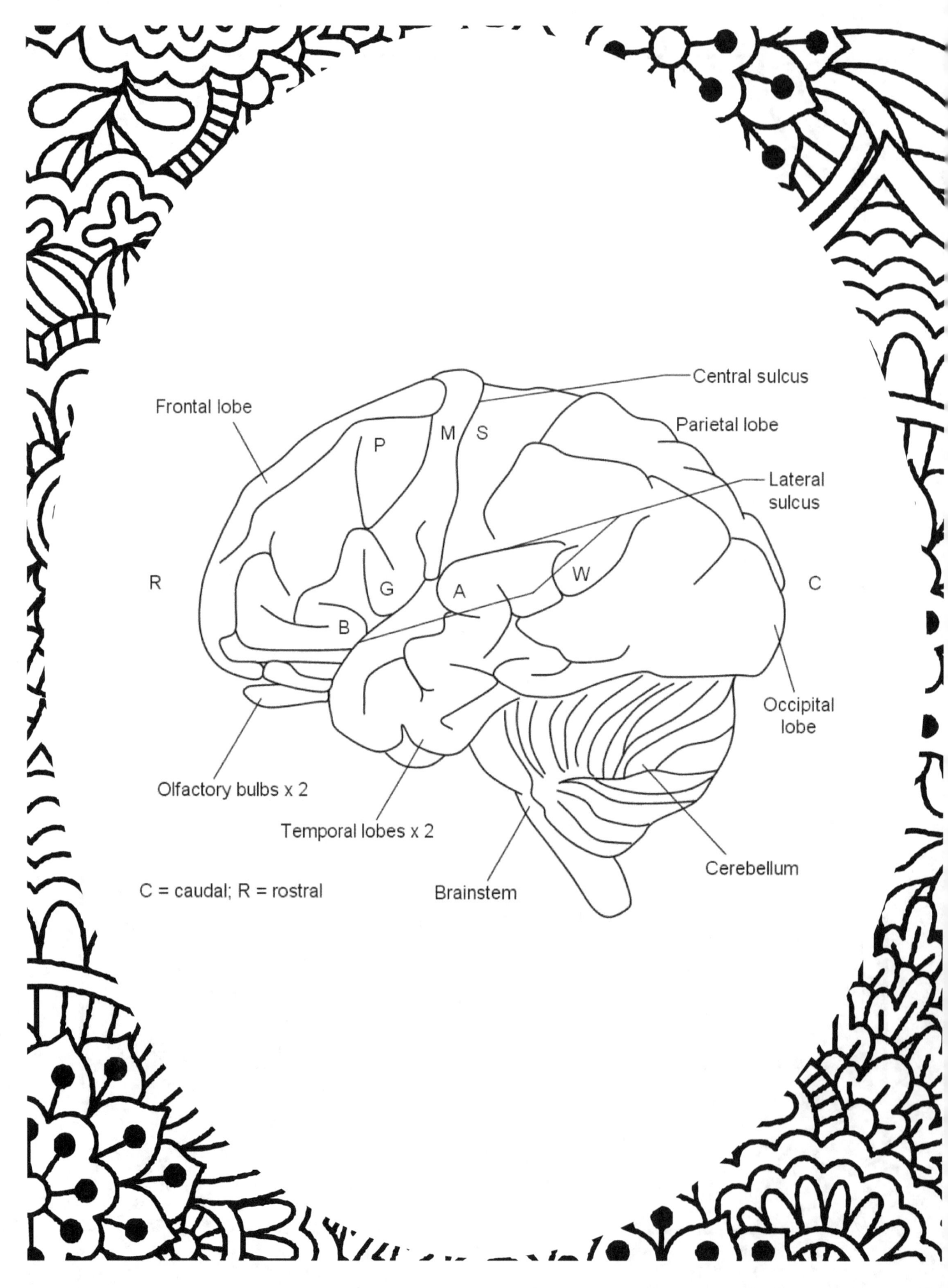

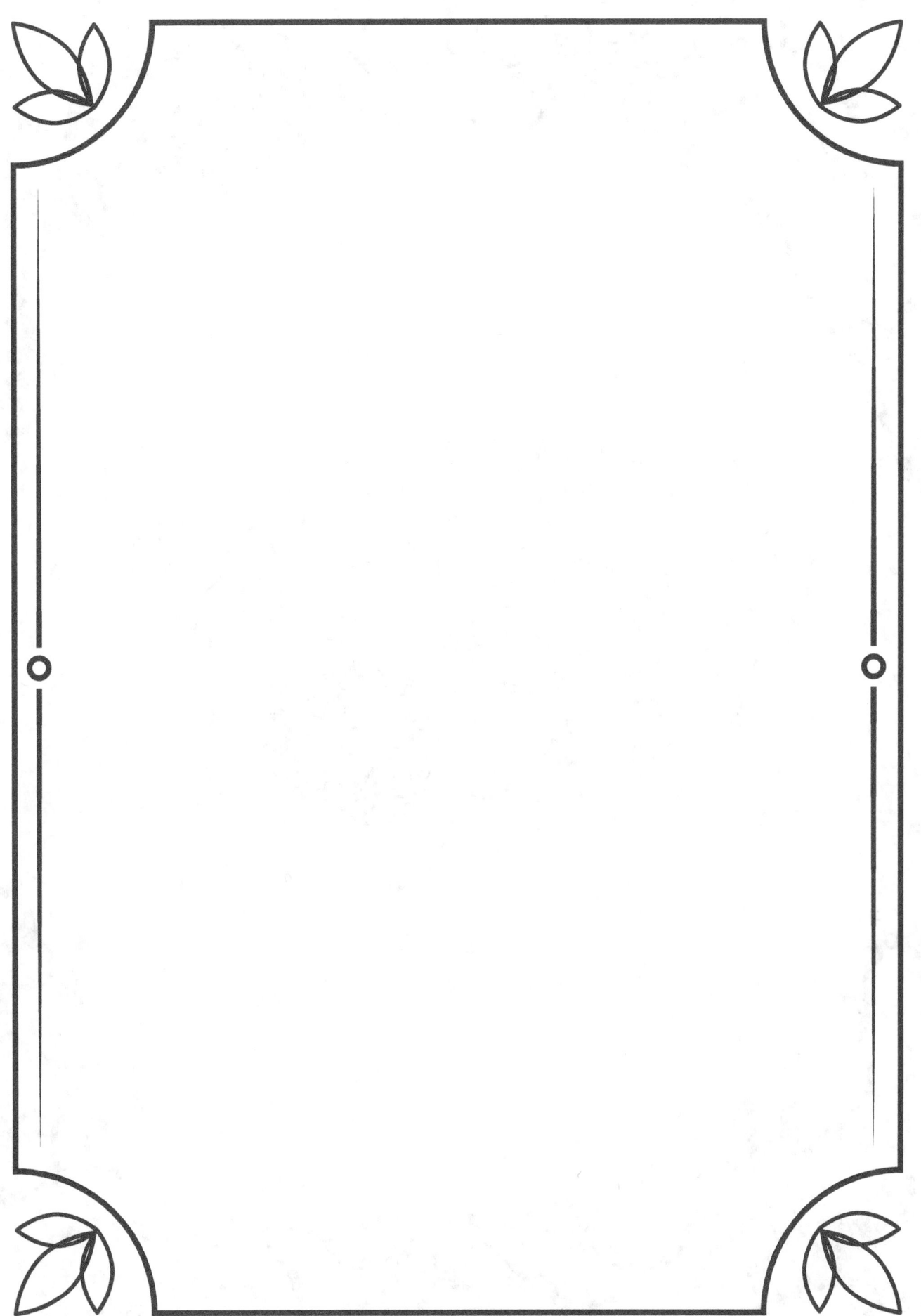

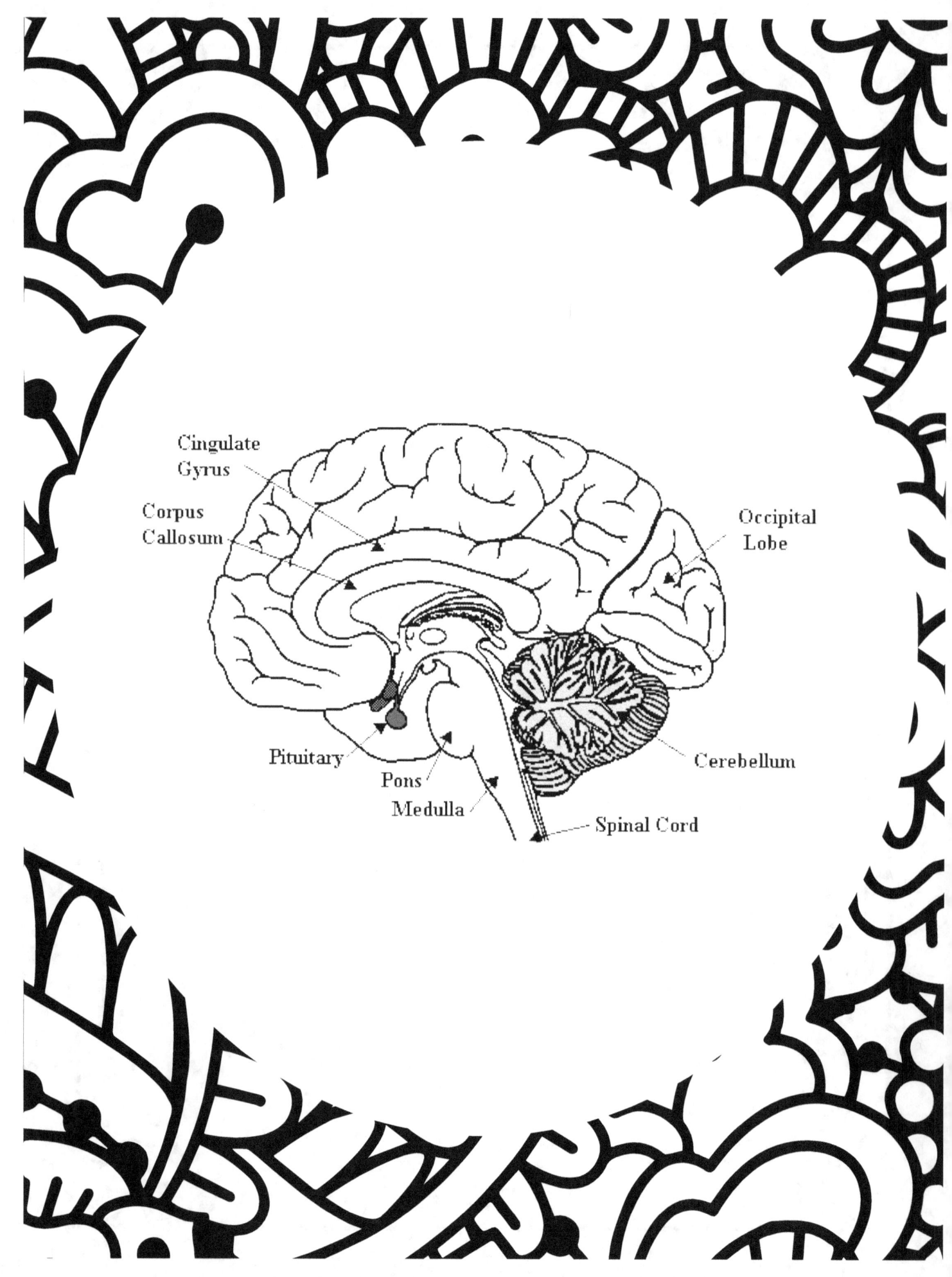

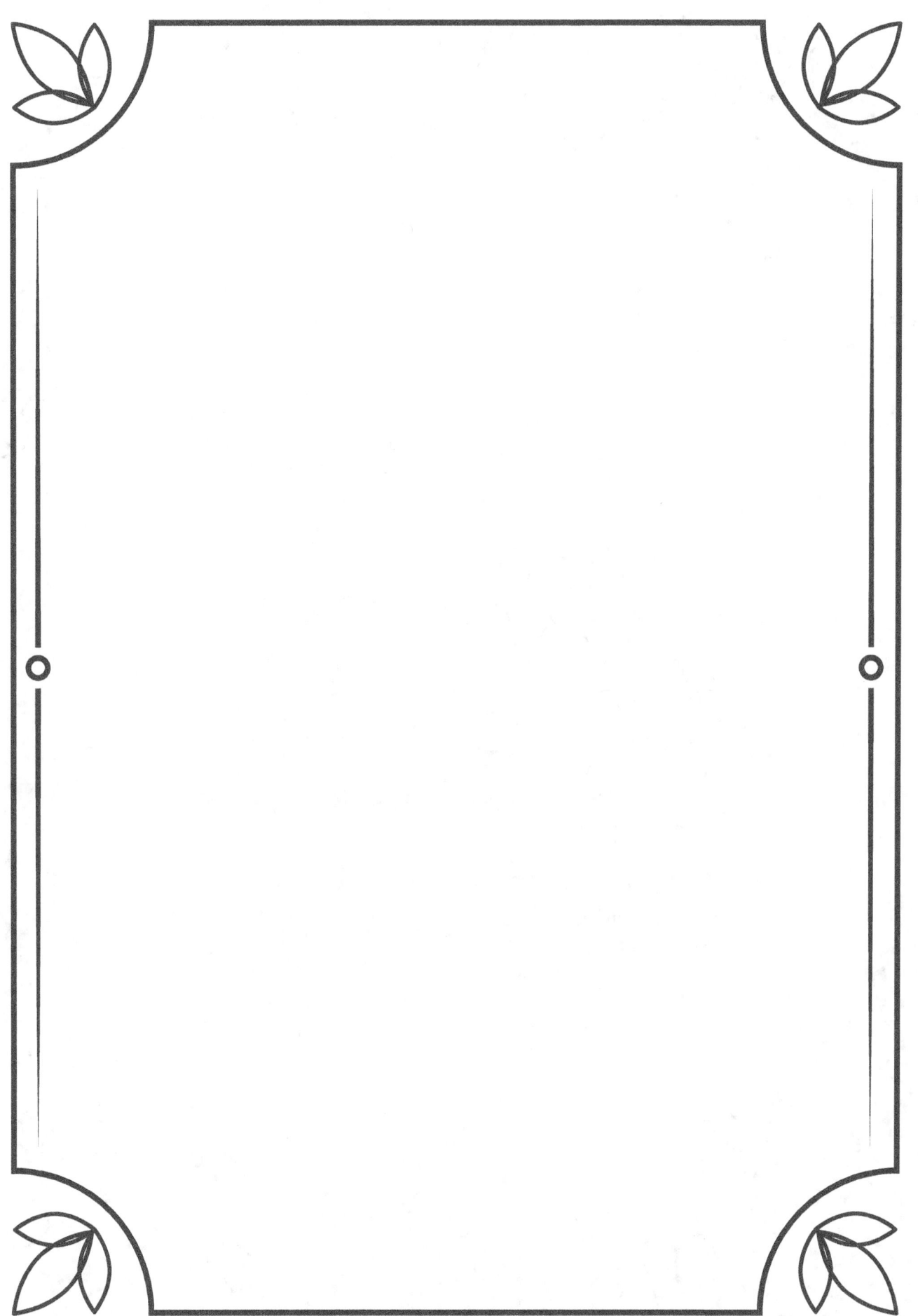

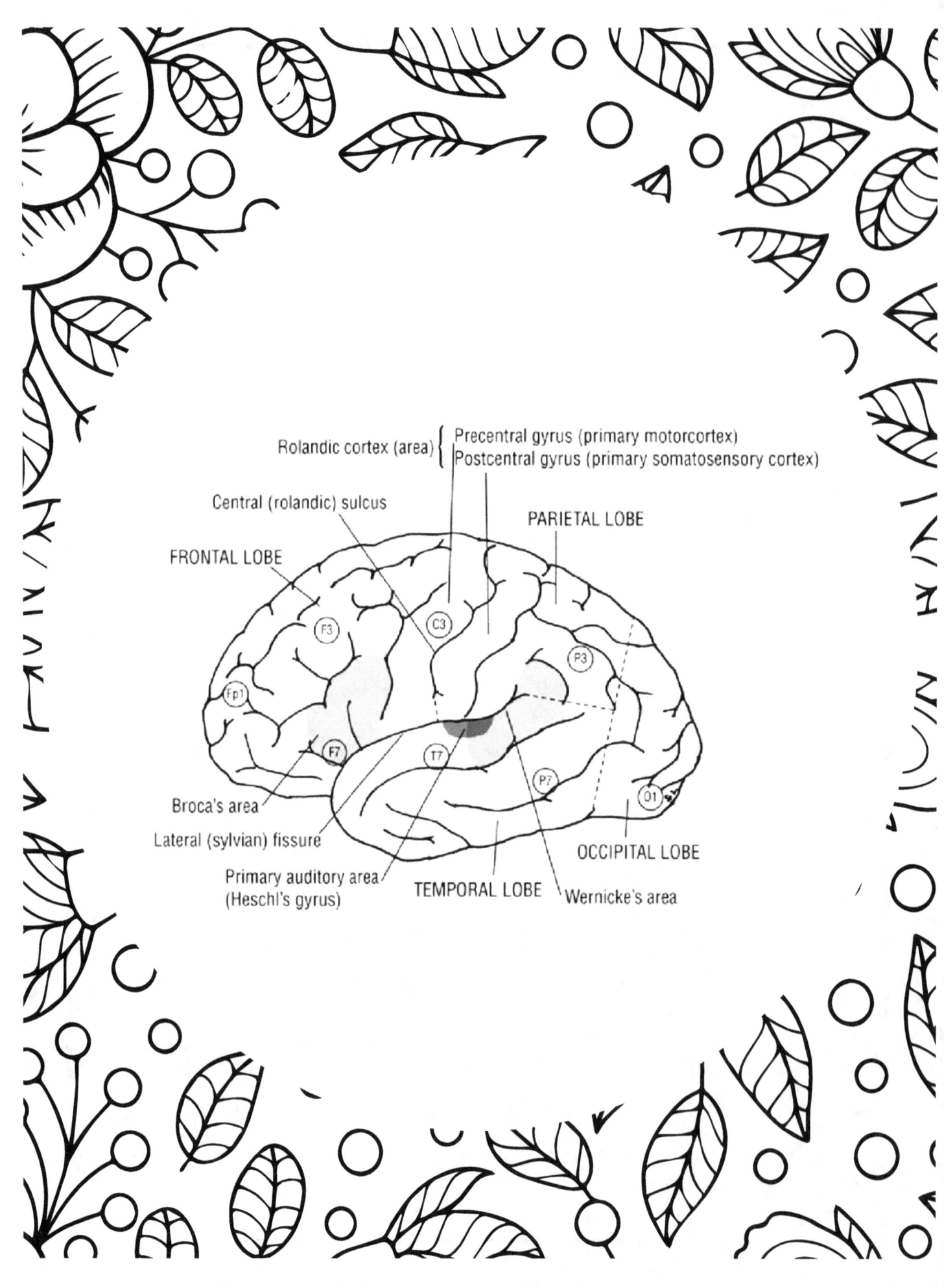

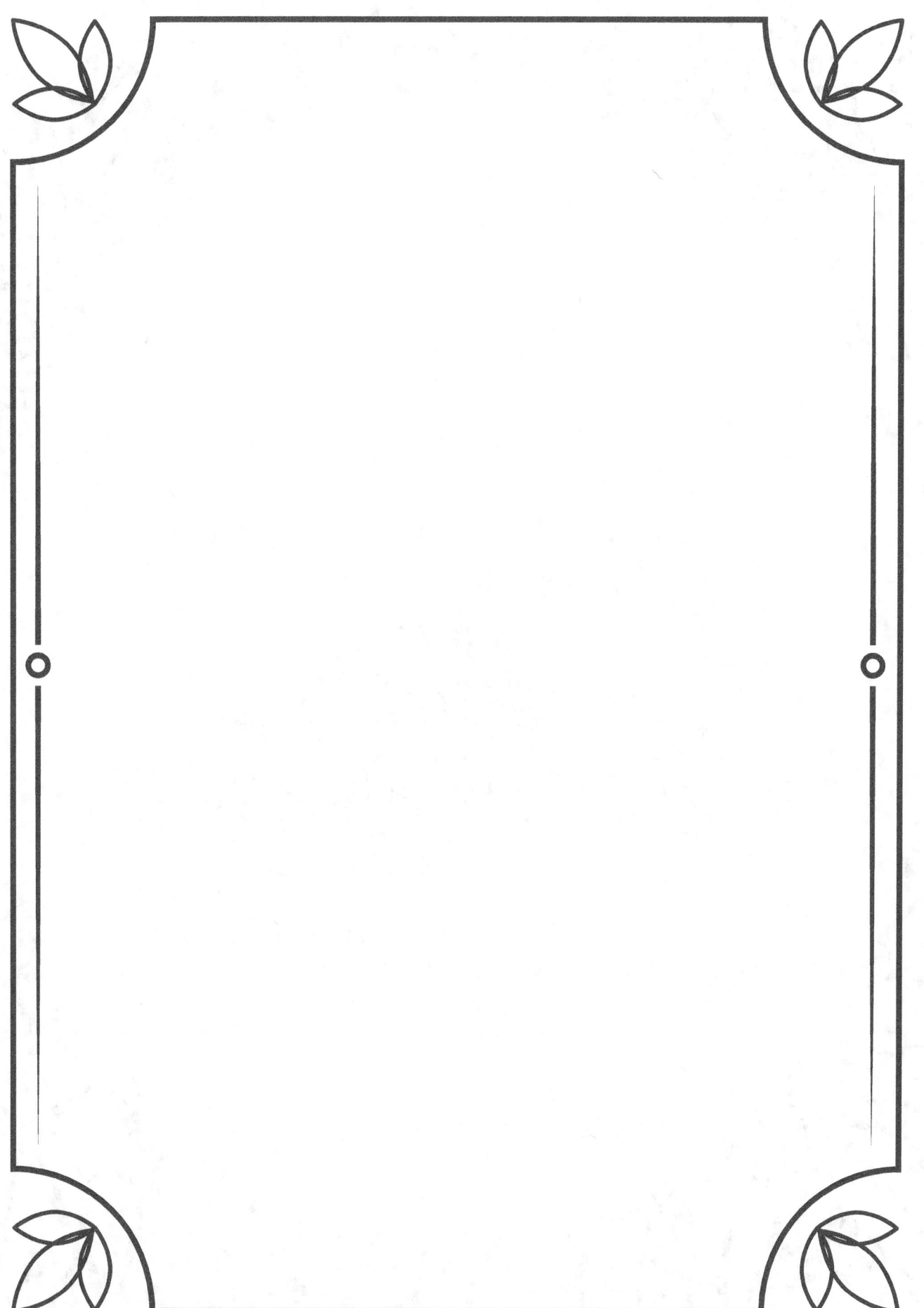

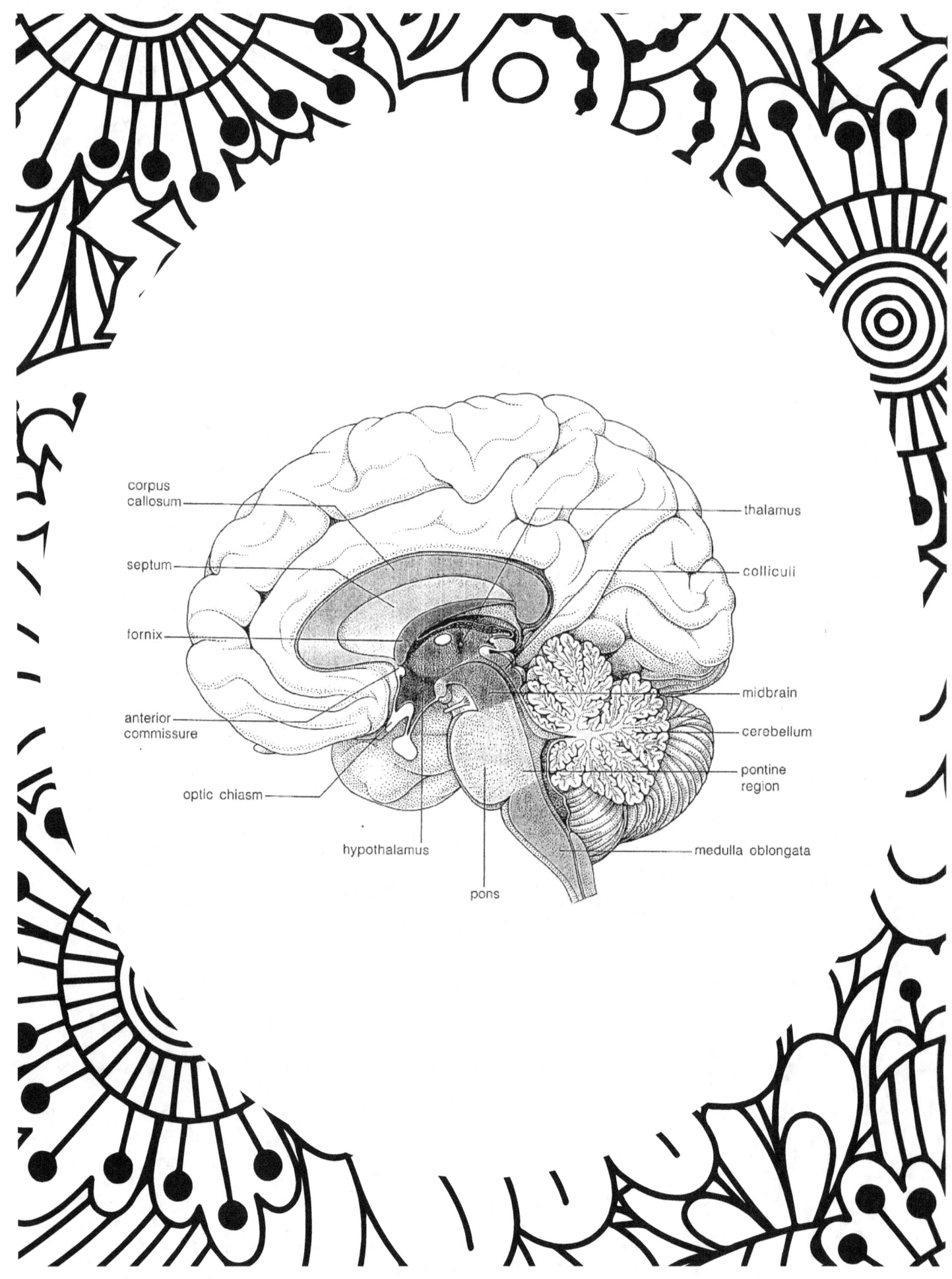

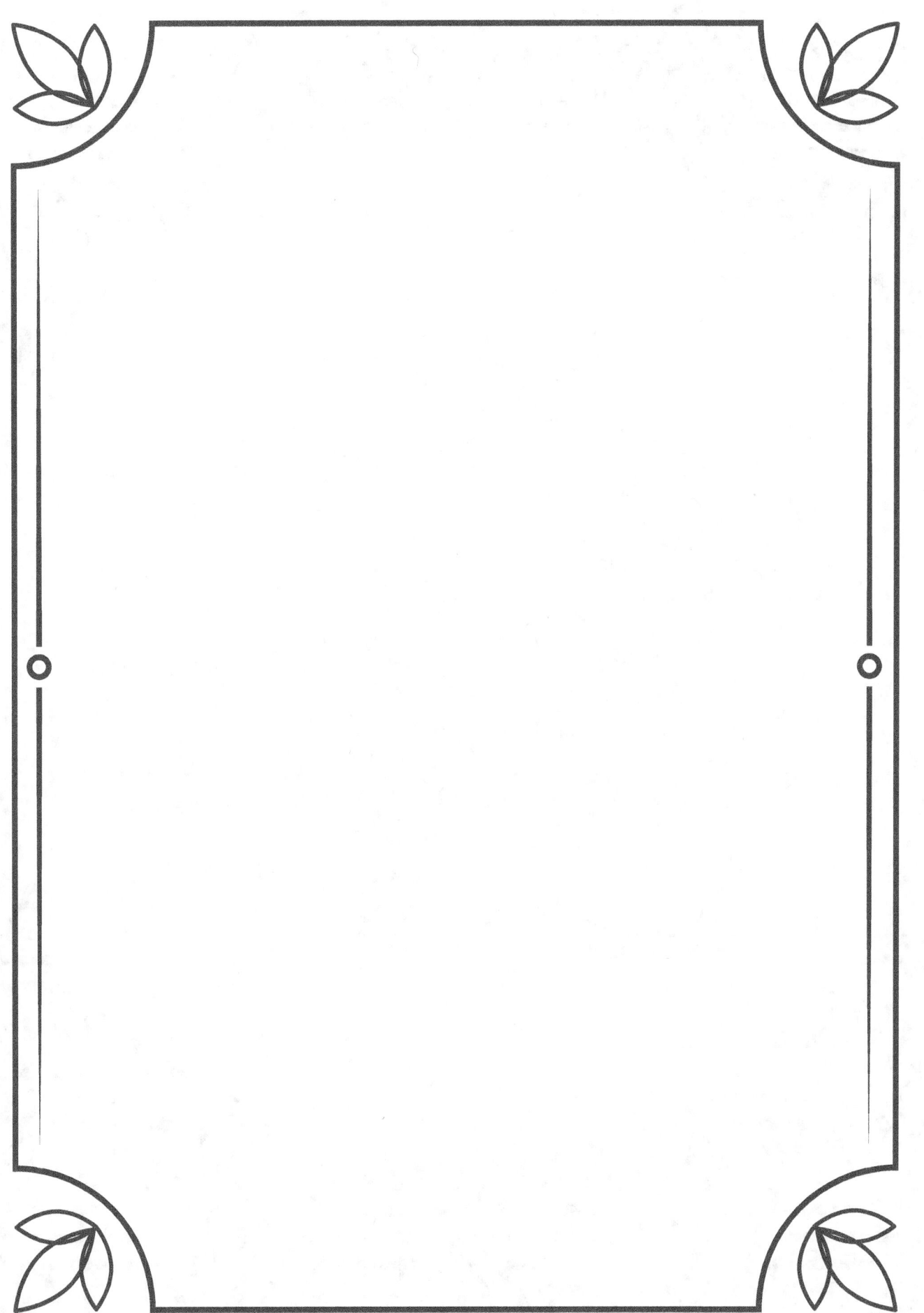

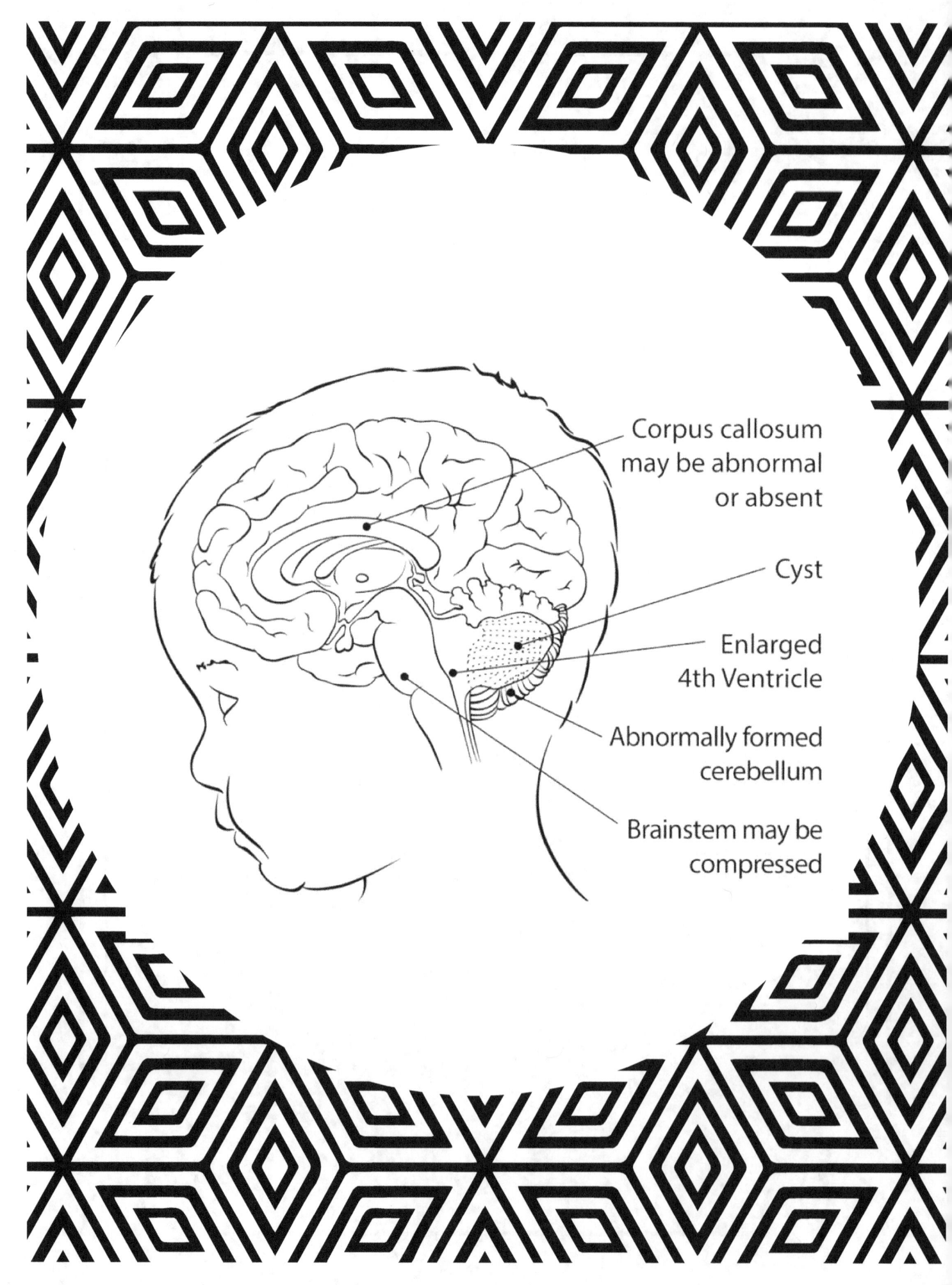

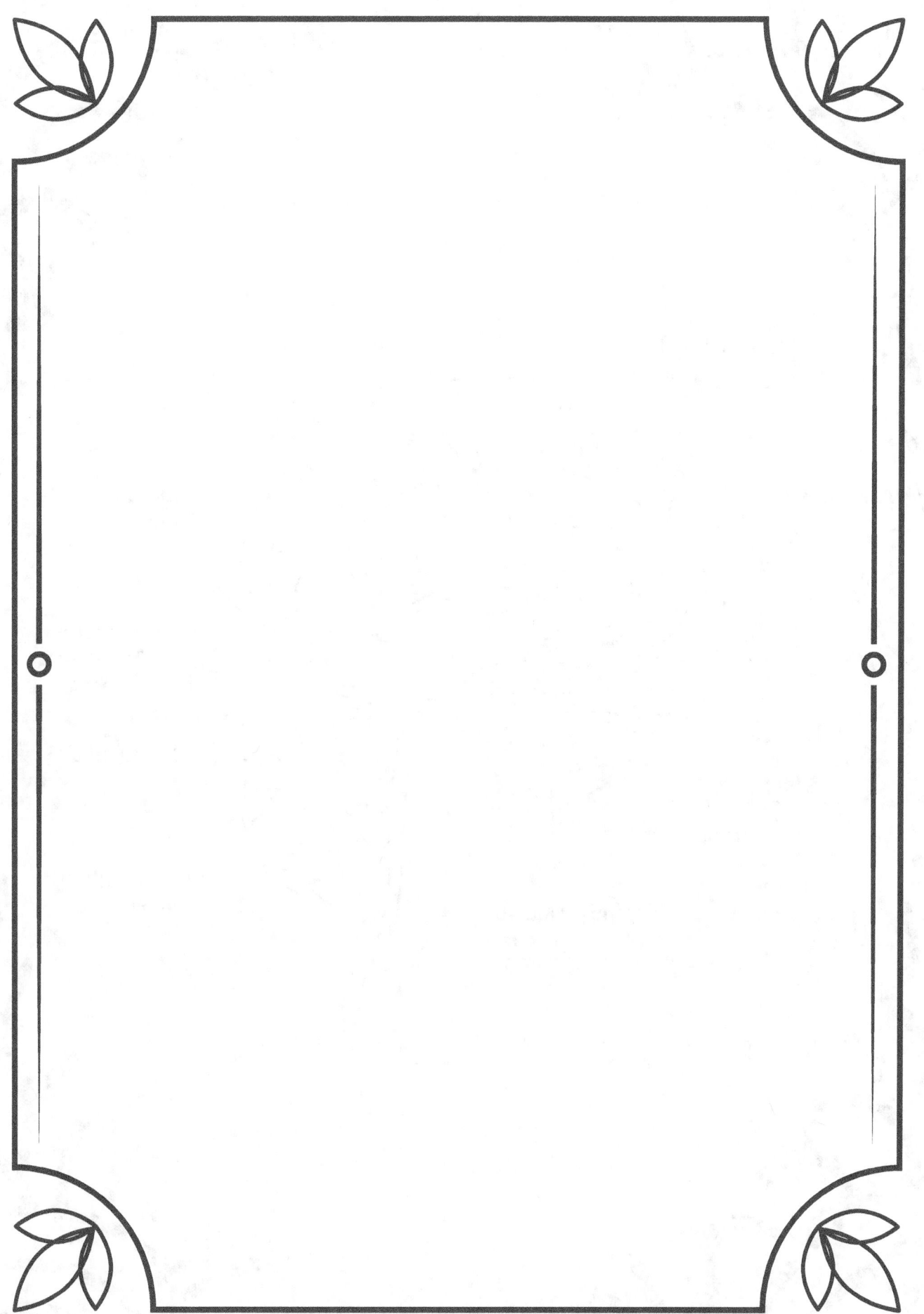

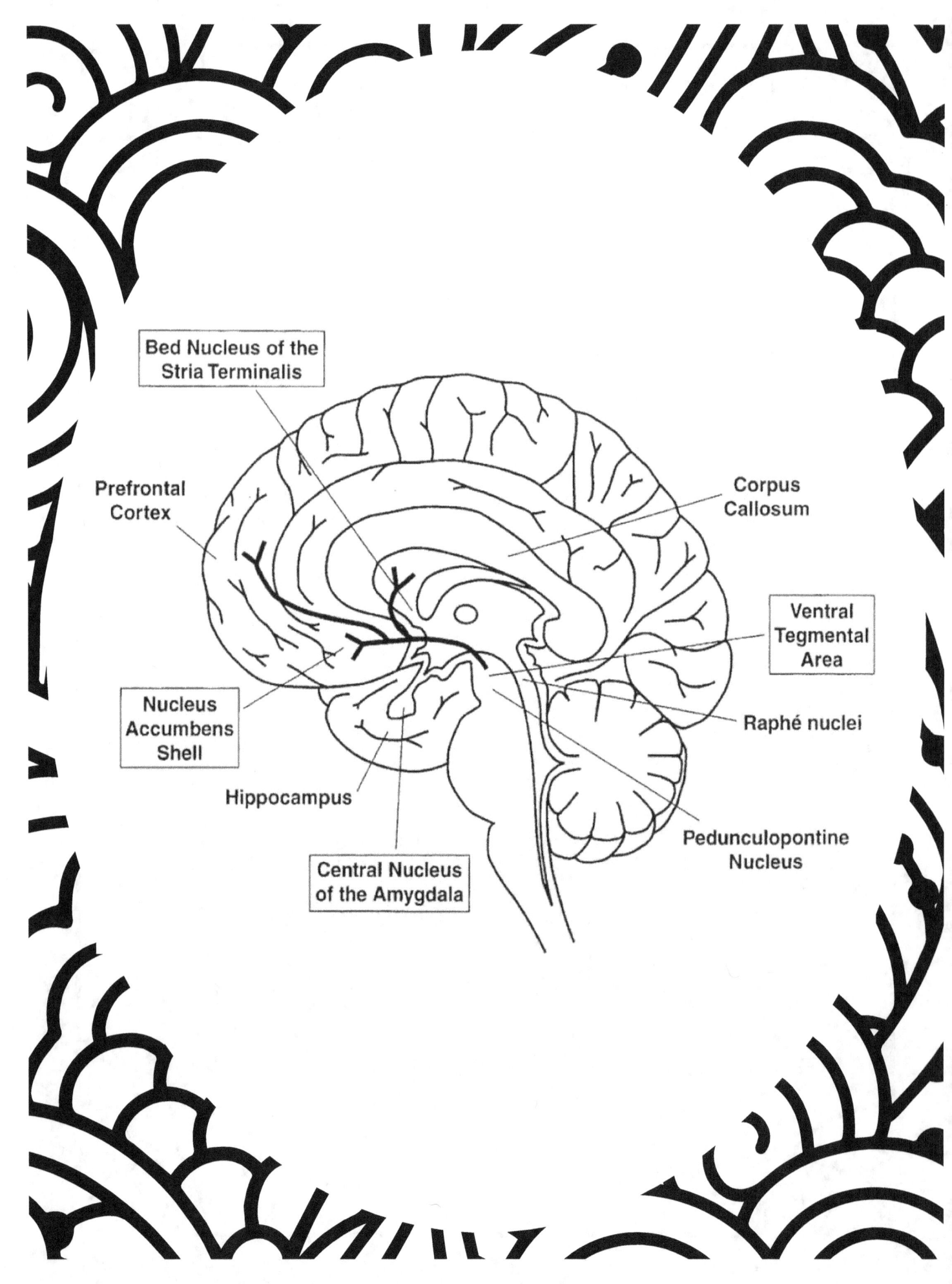

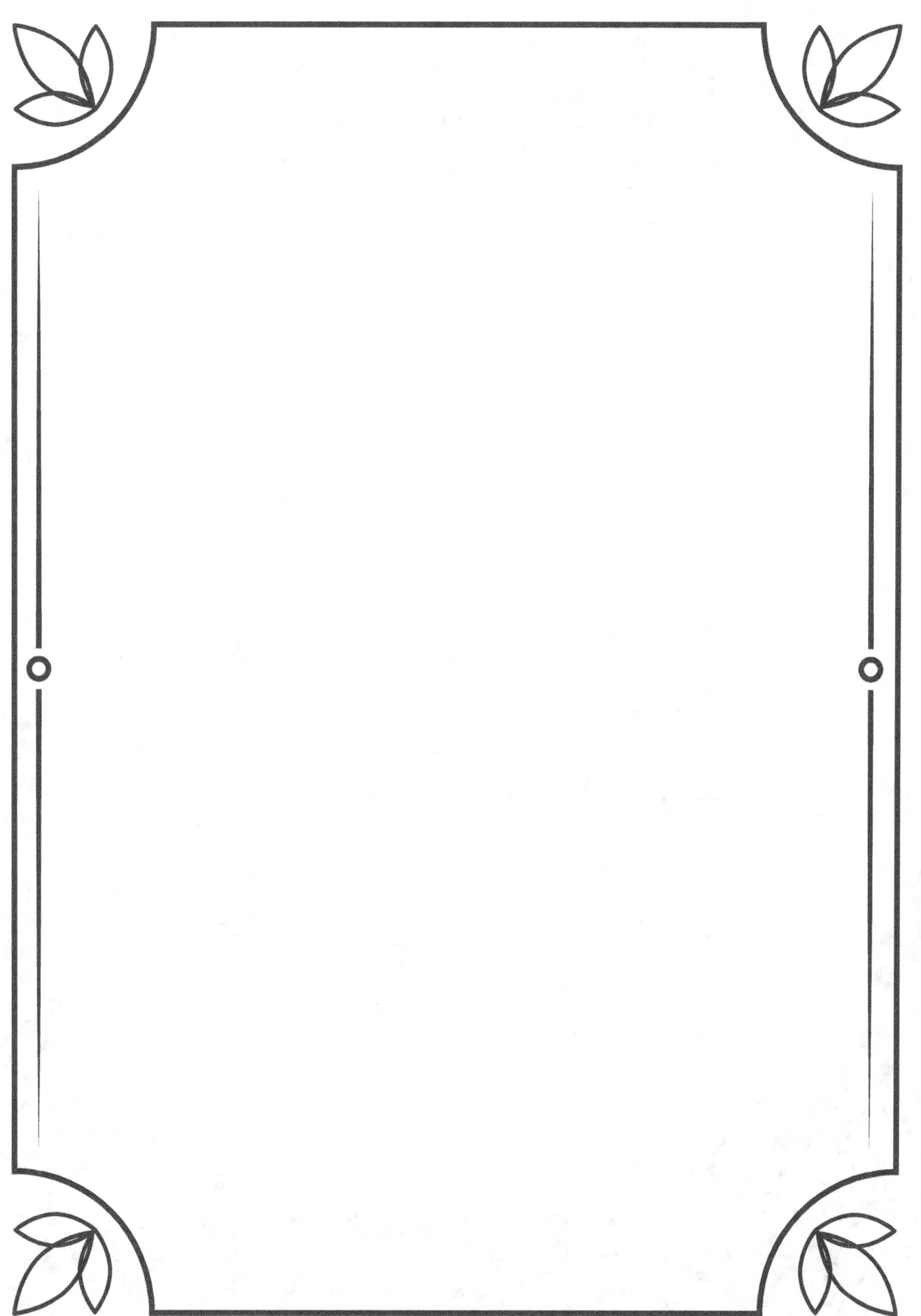

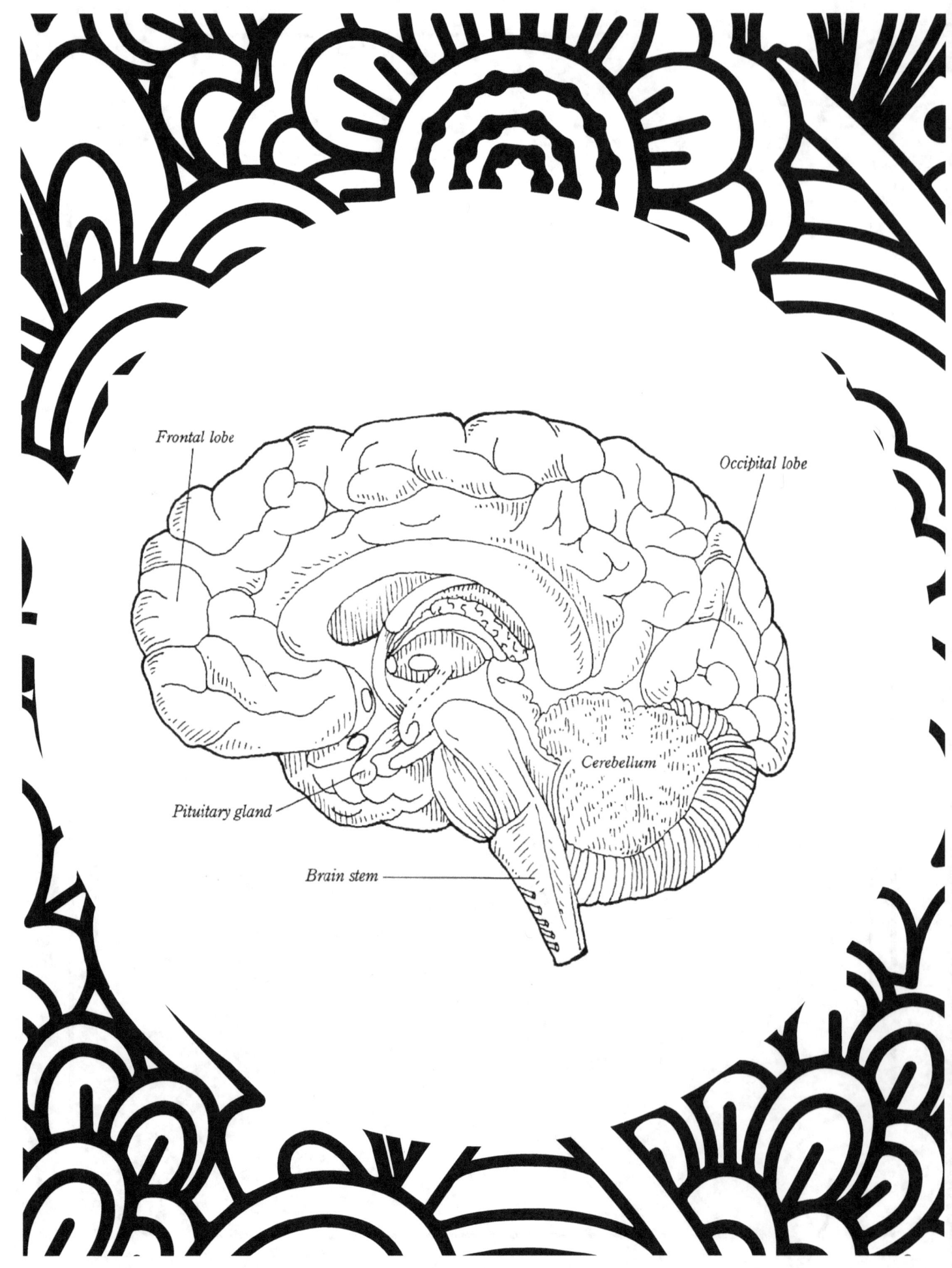

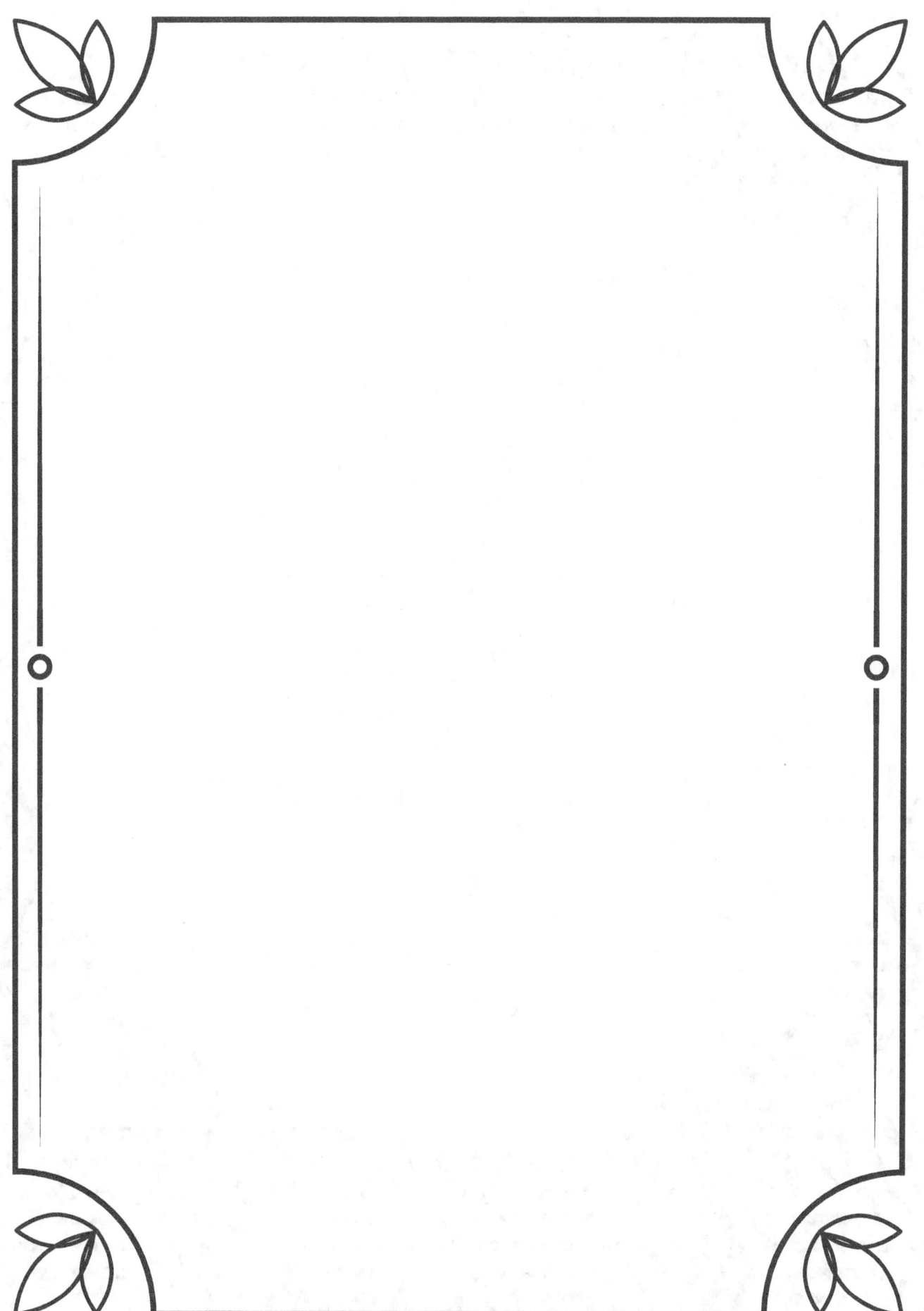

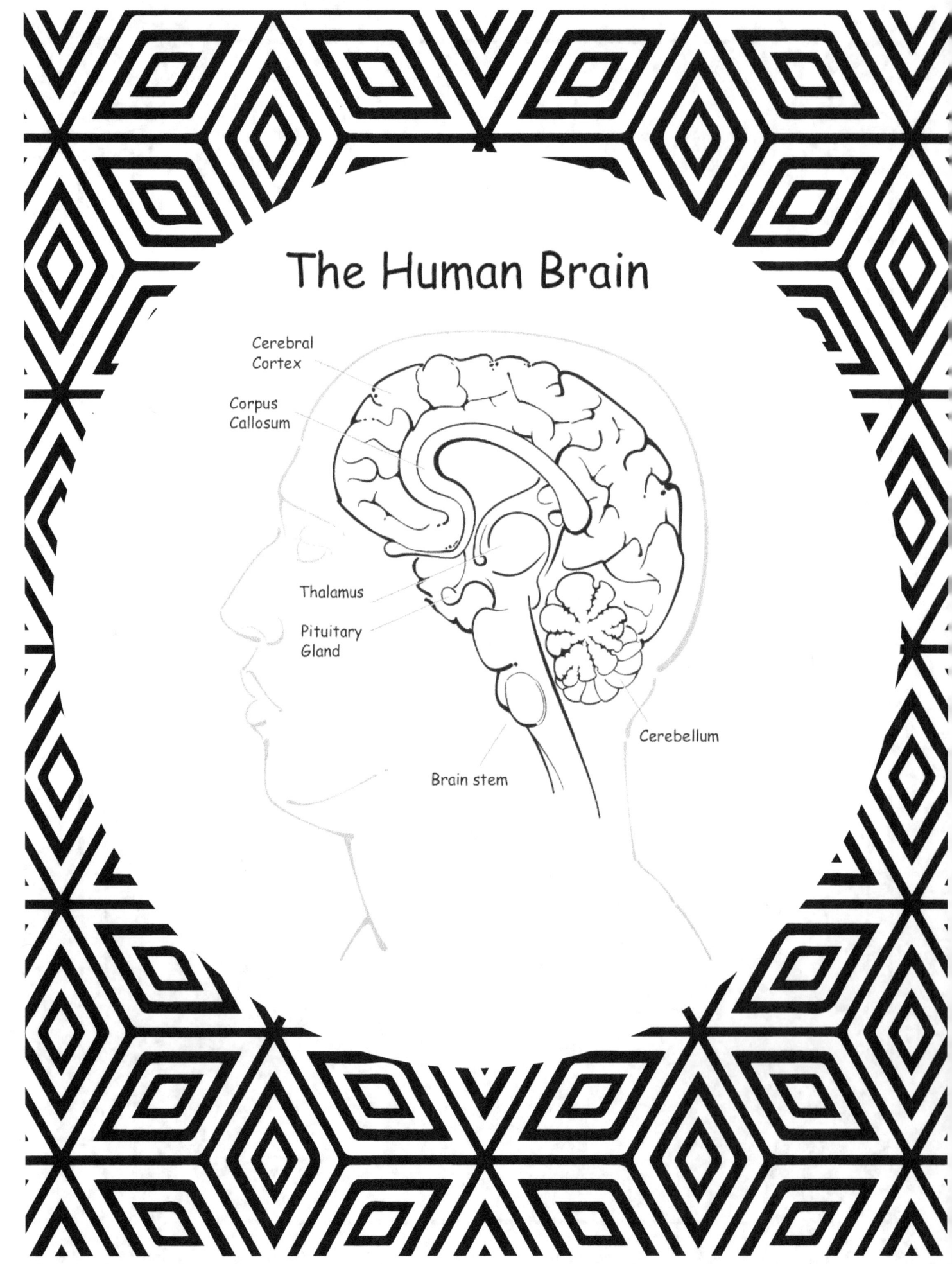

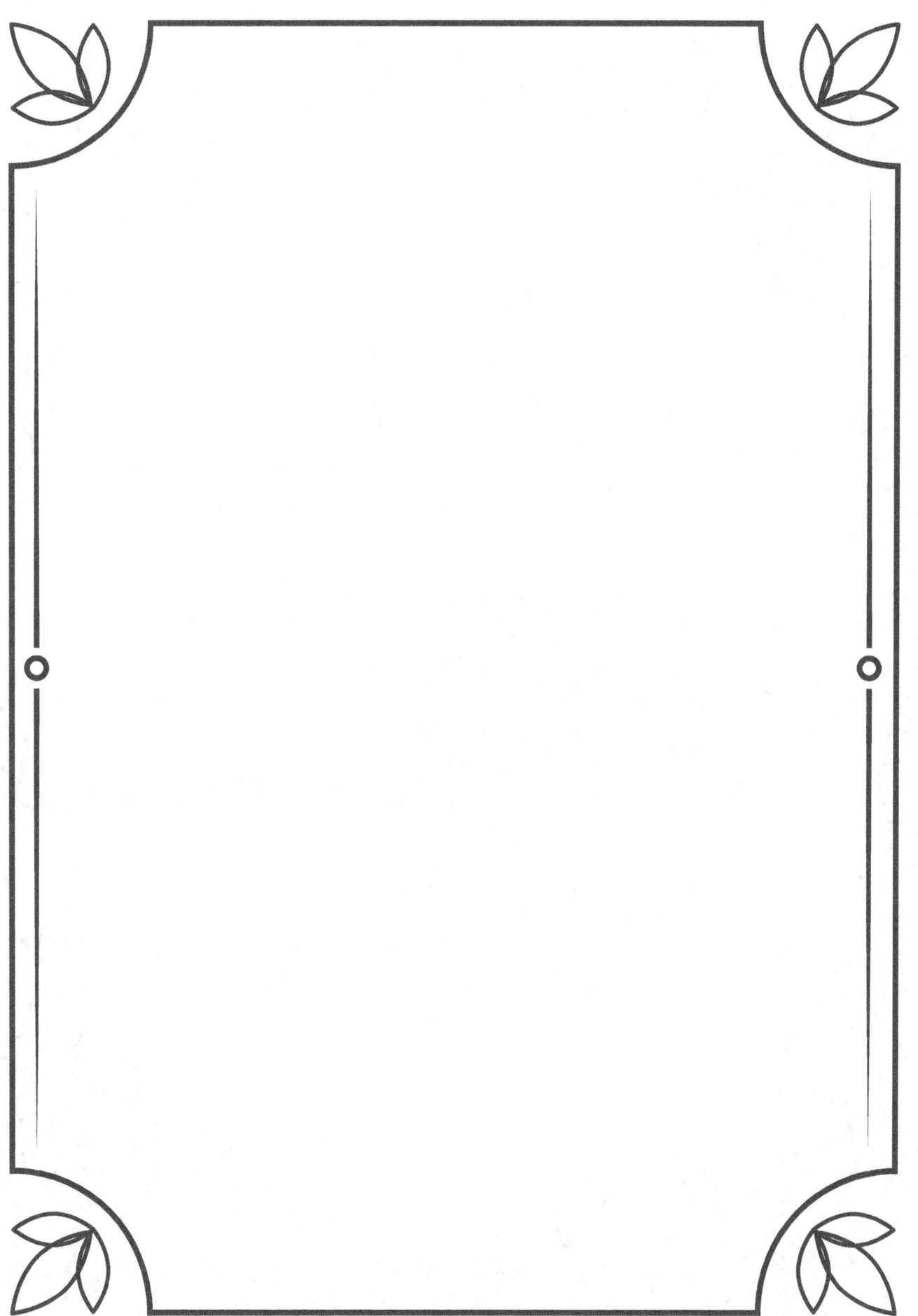

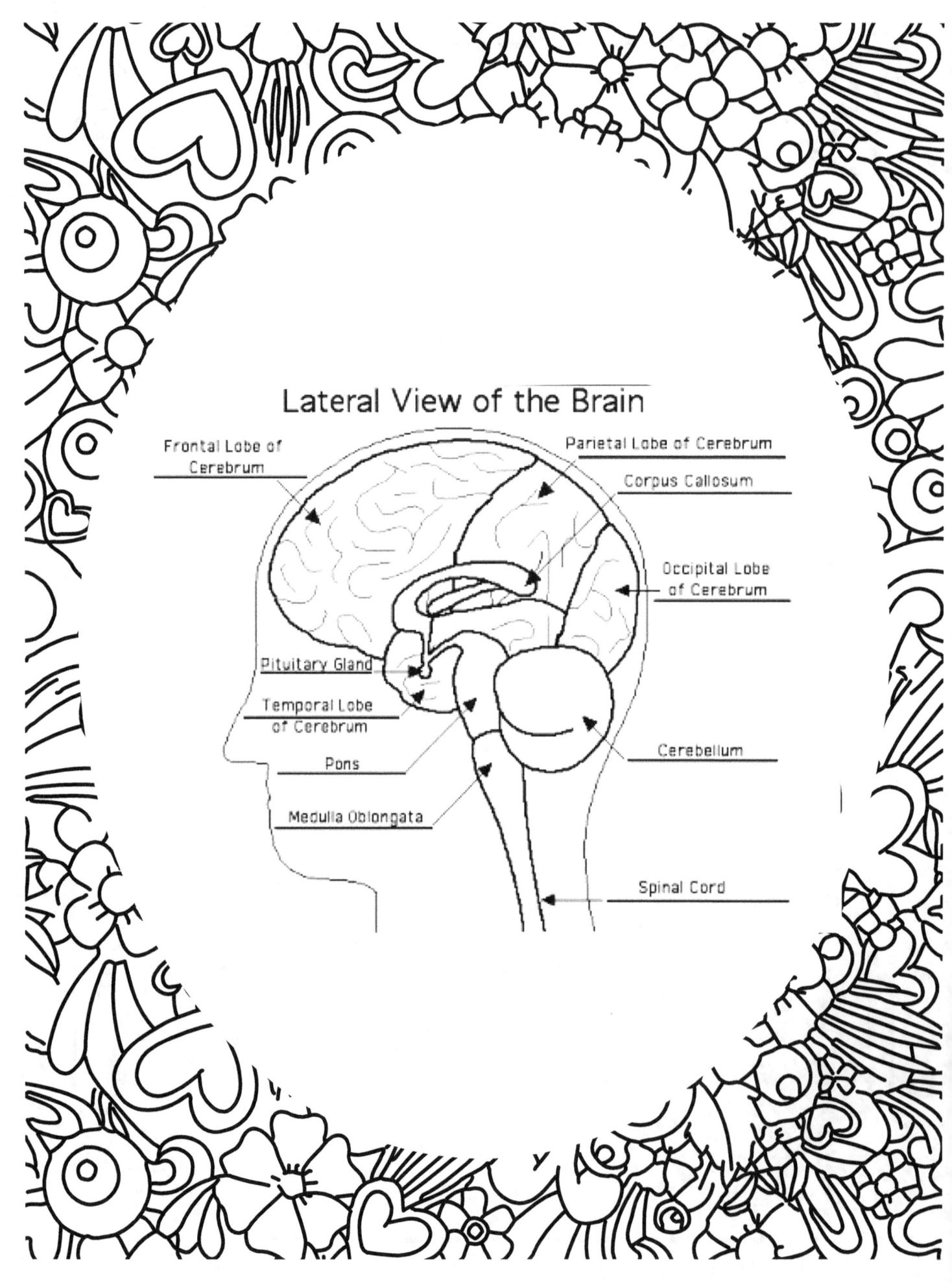

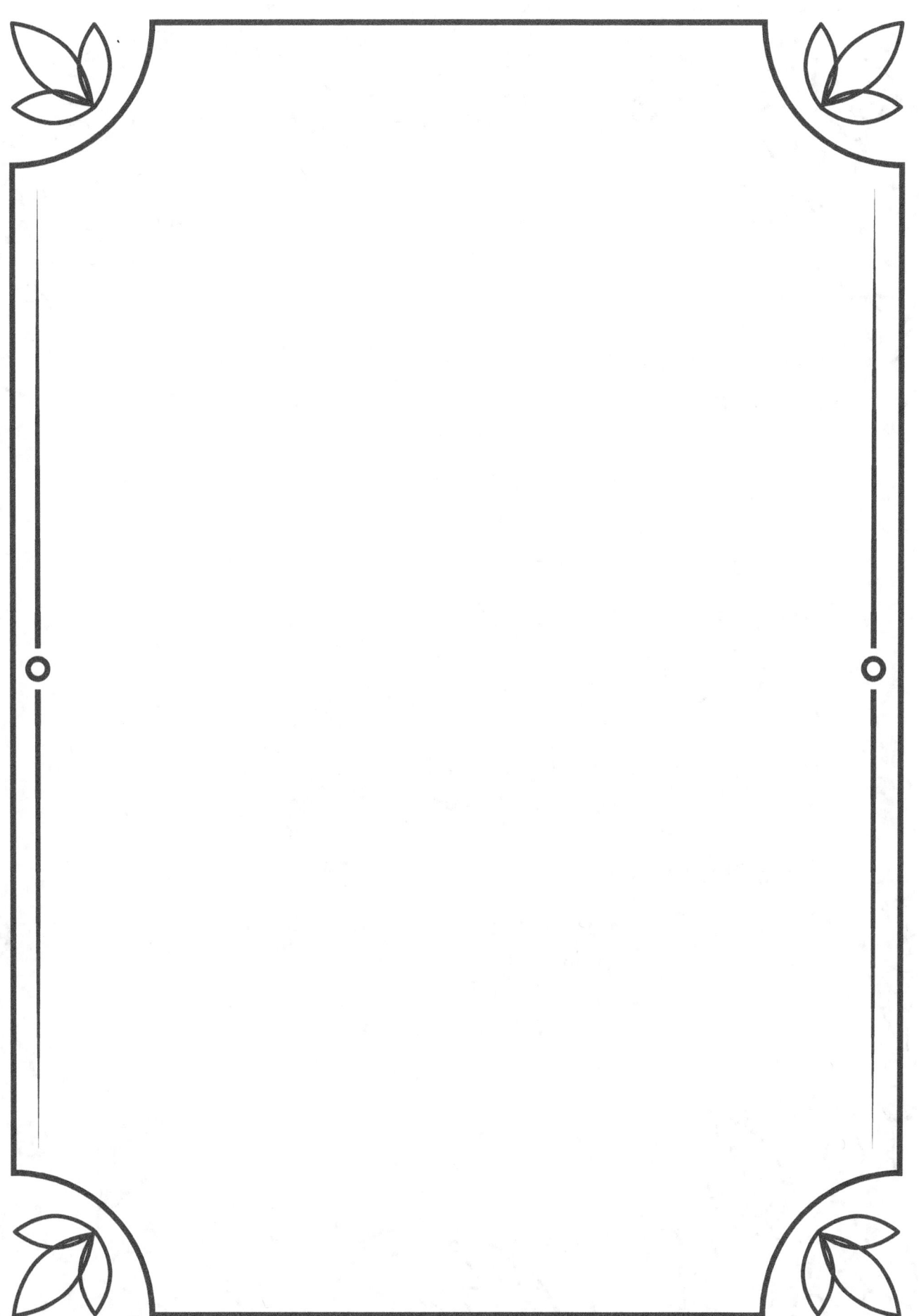

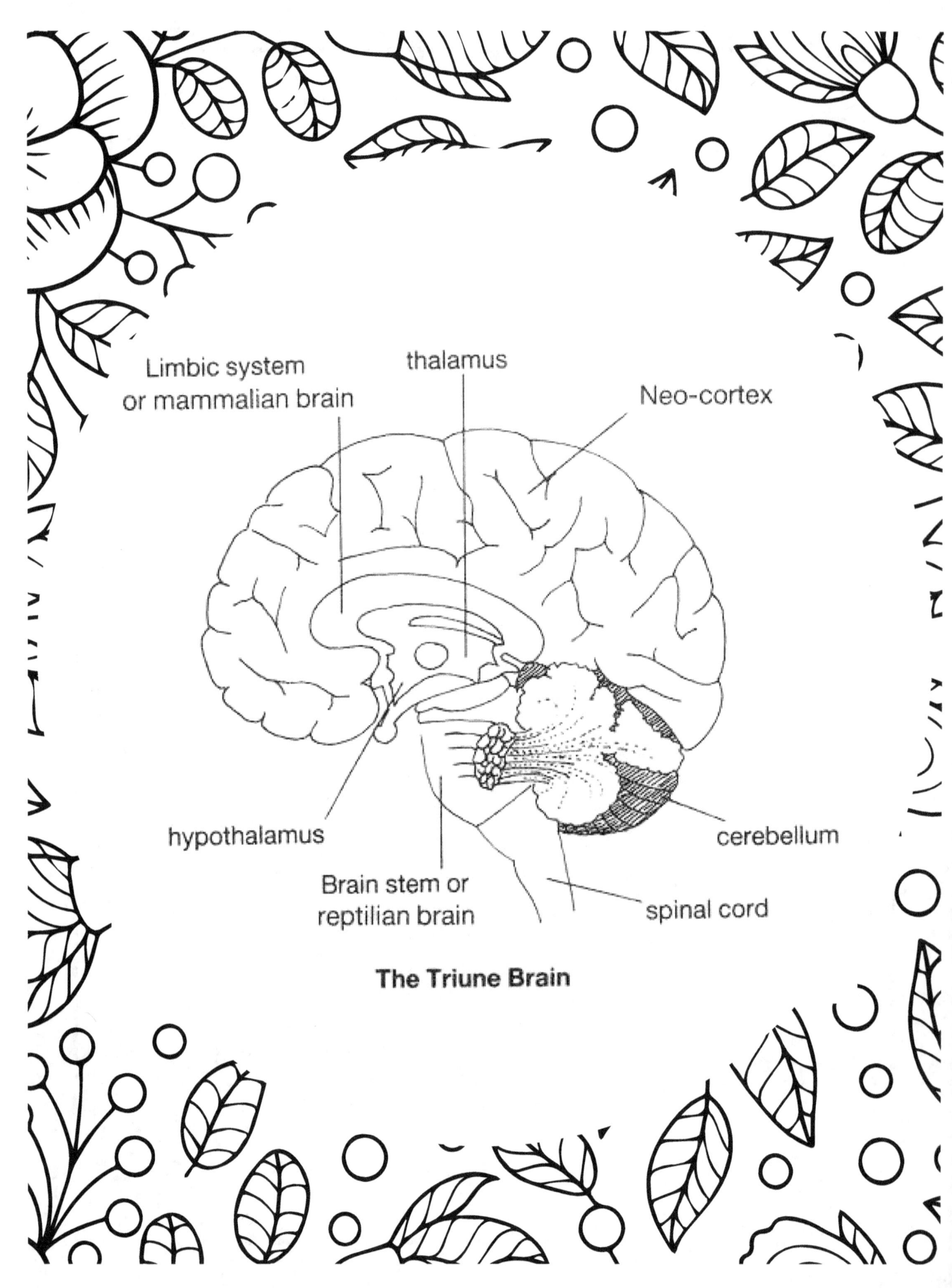

The Triune Brain

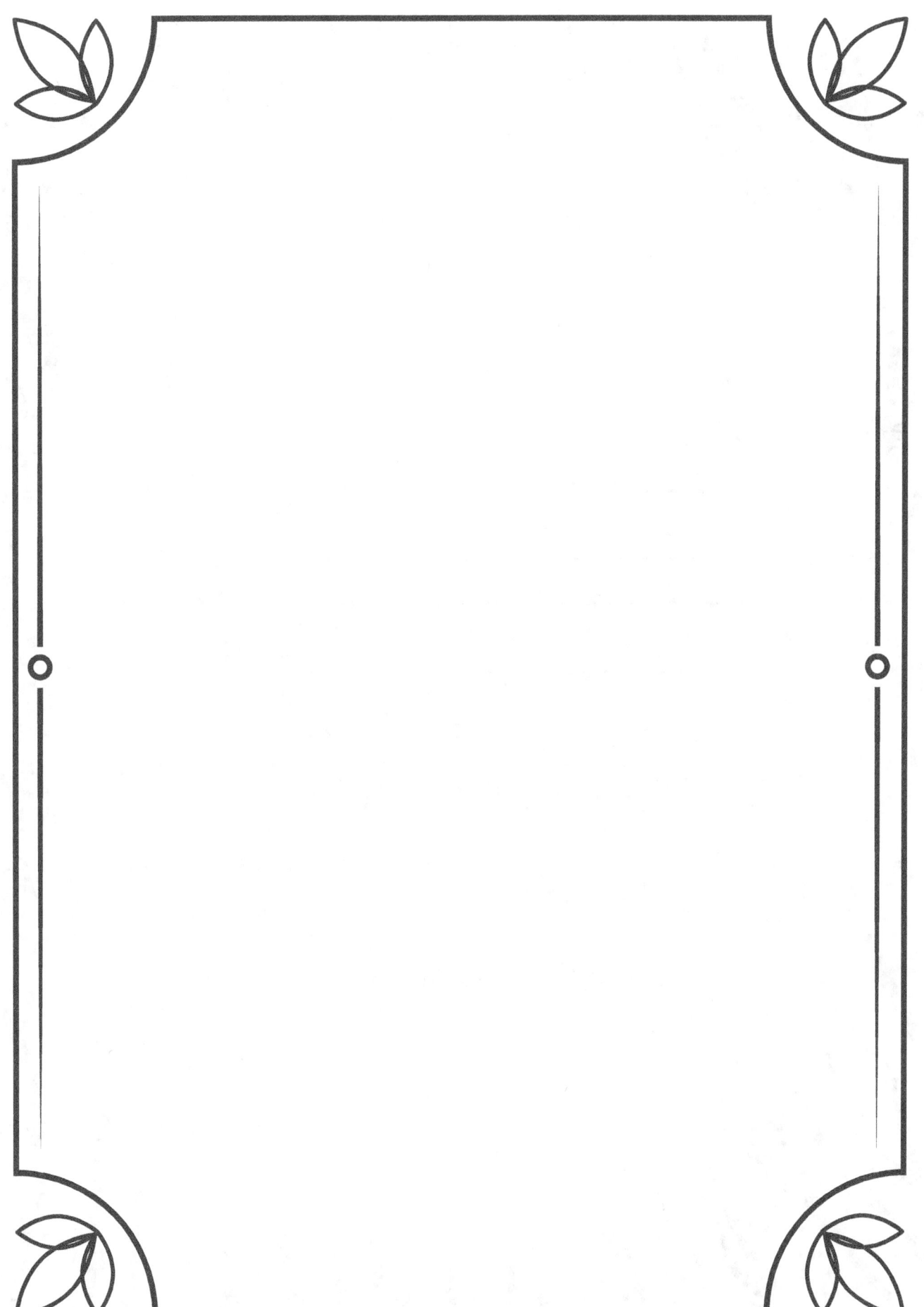

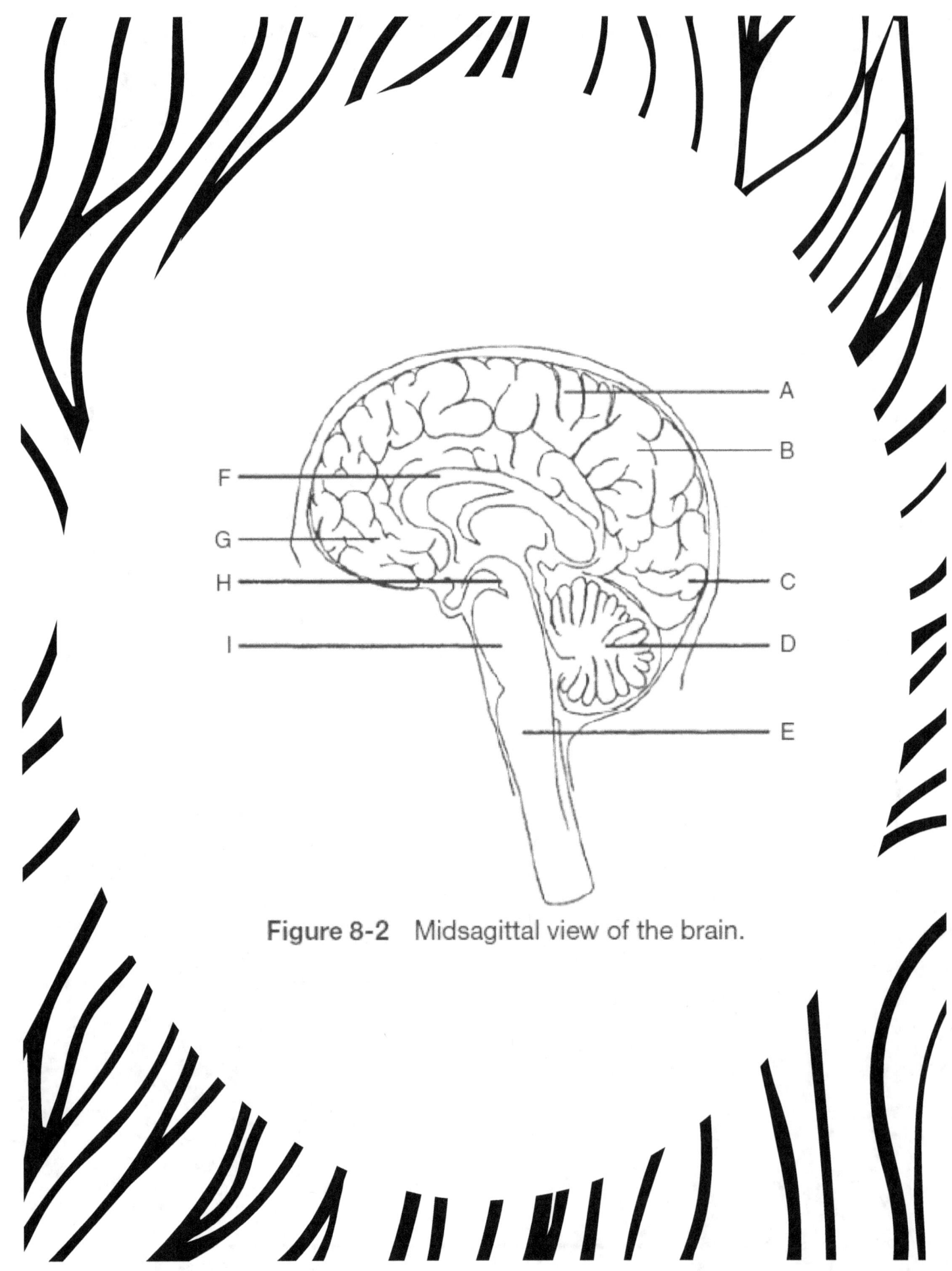

Figure 8-2 Midsagittal view of the brain.

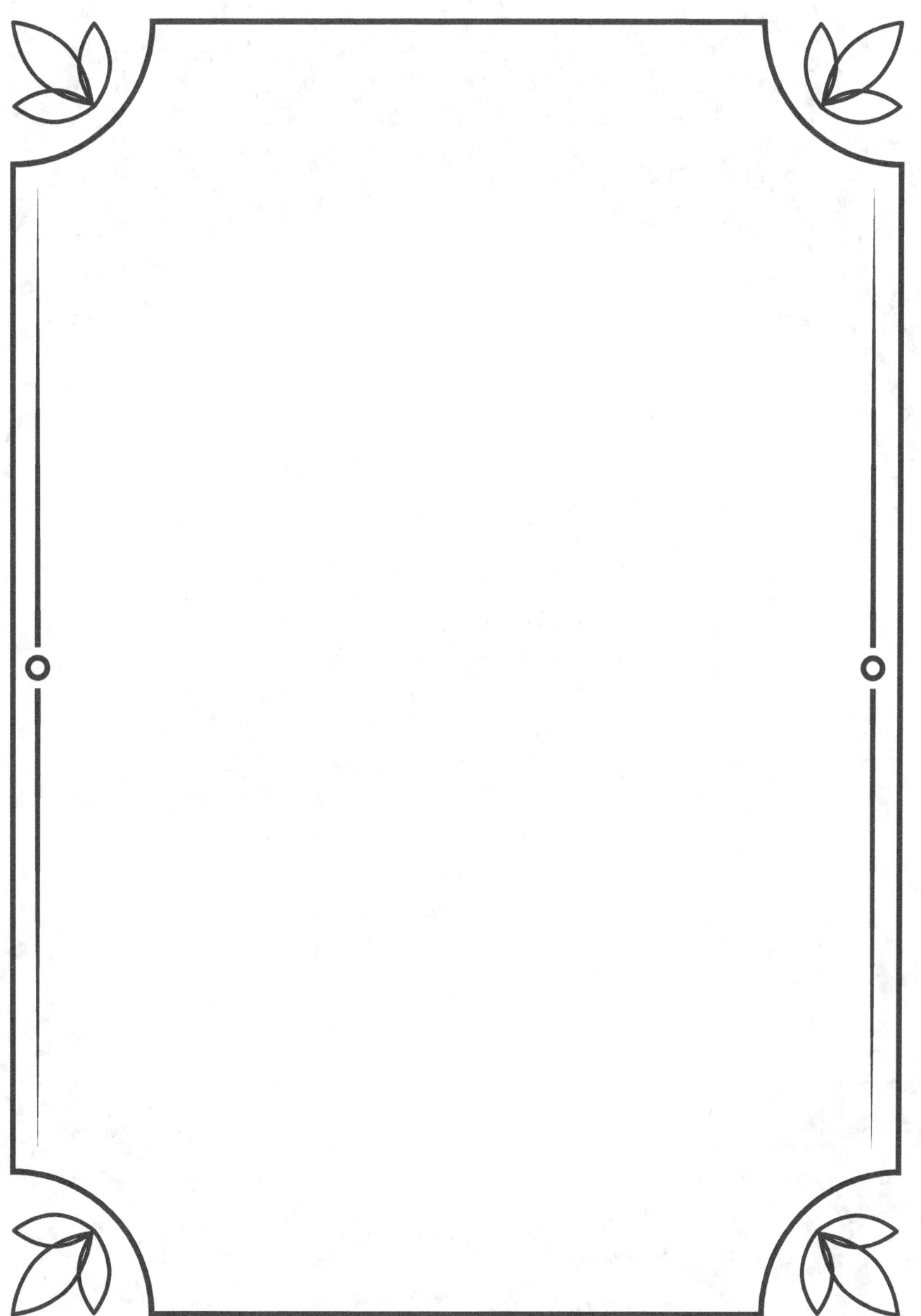

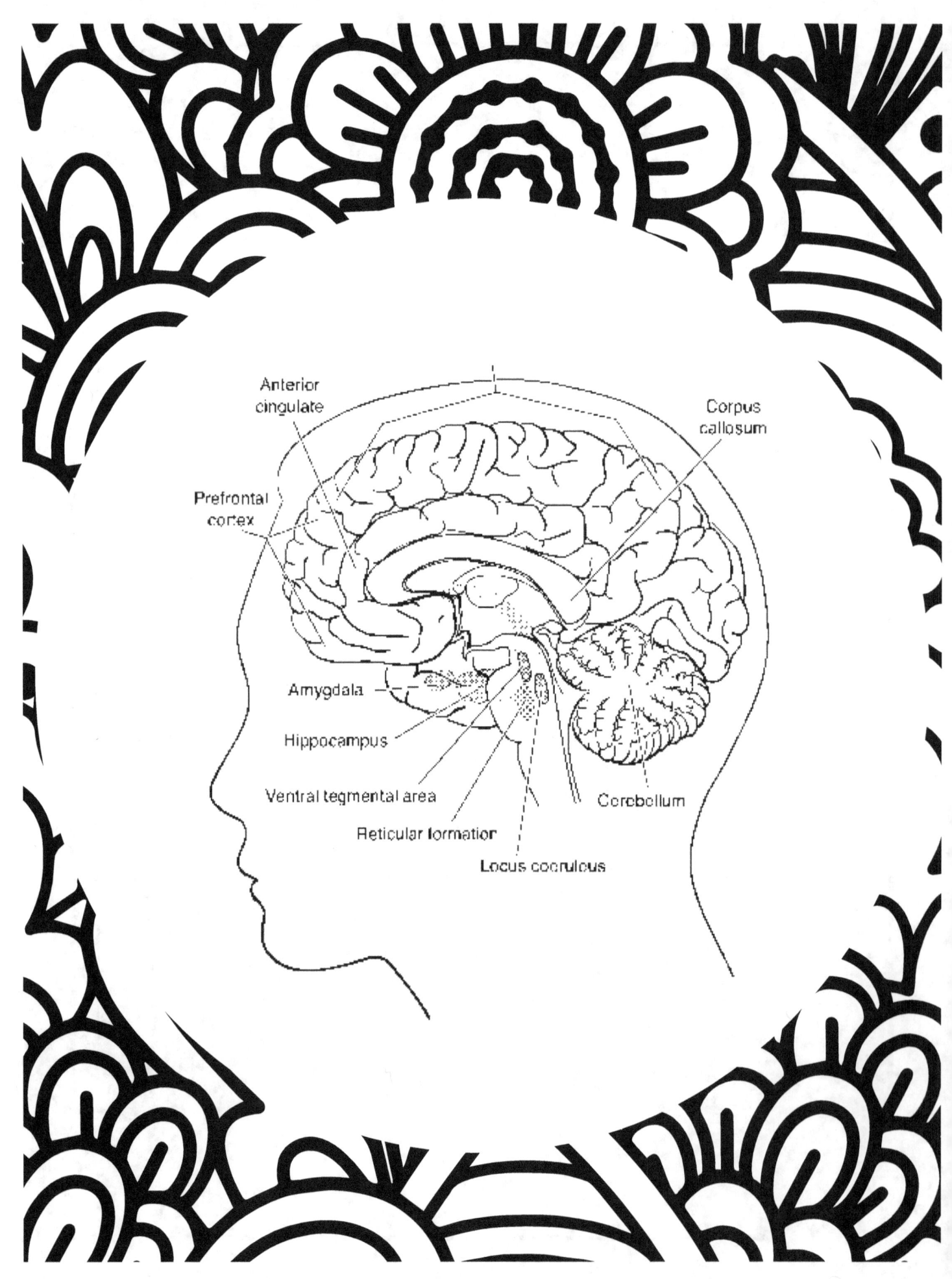

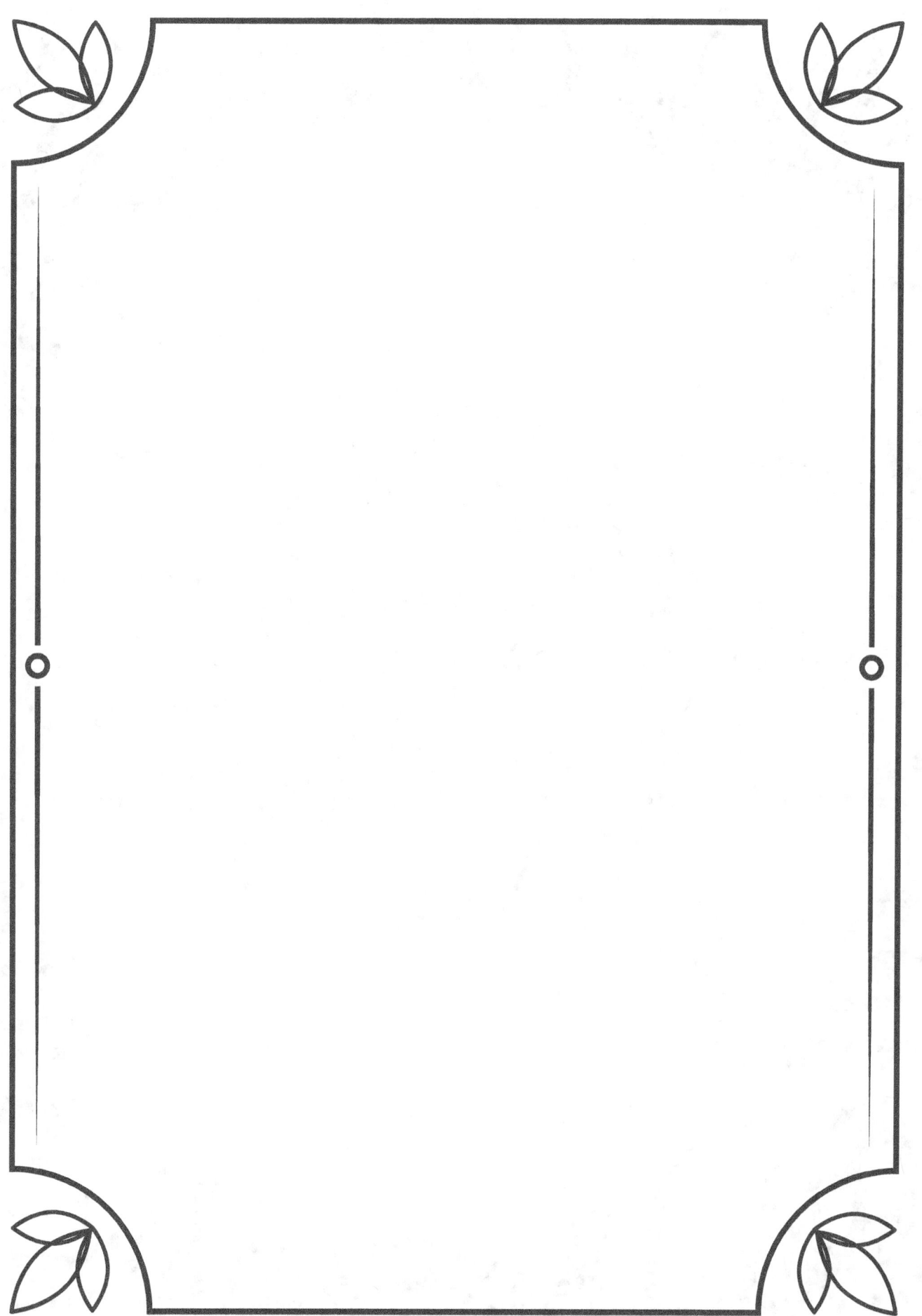

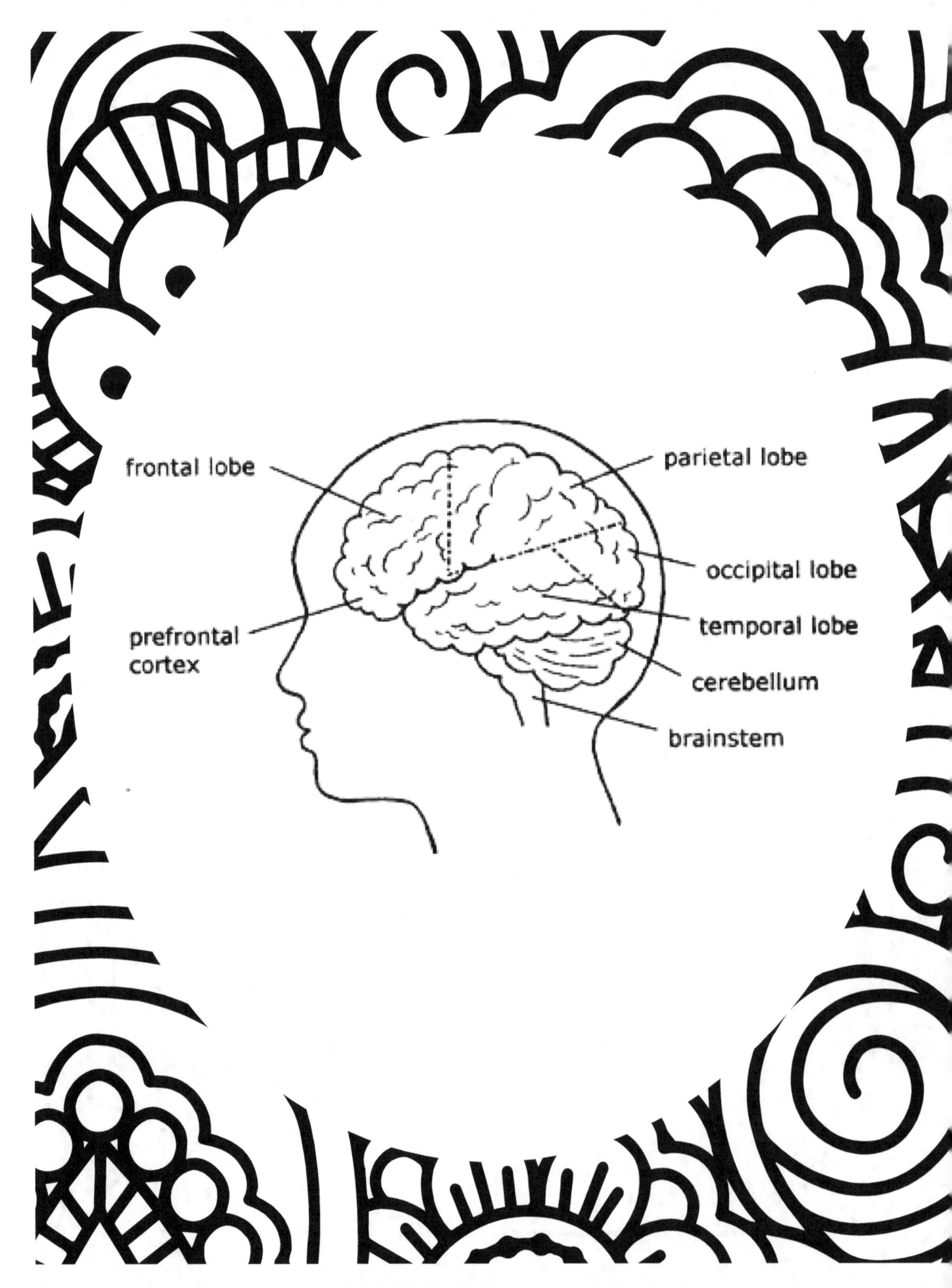

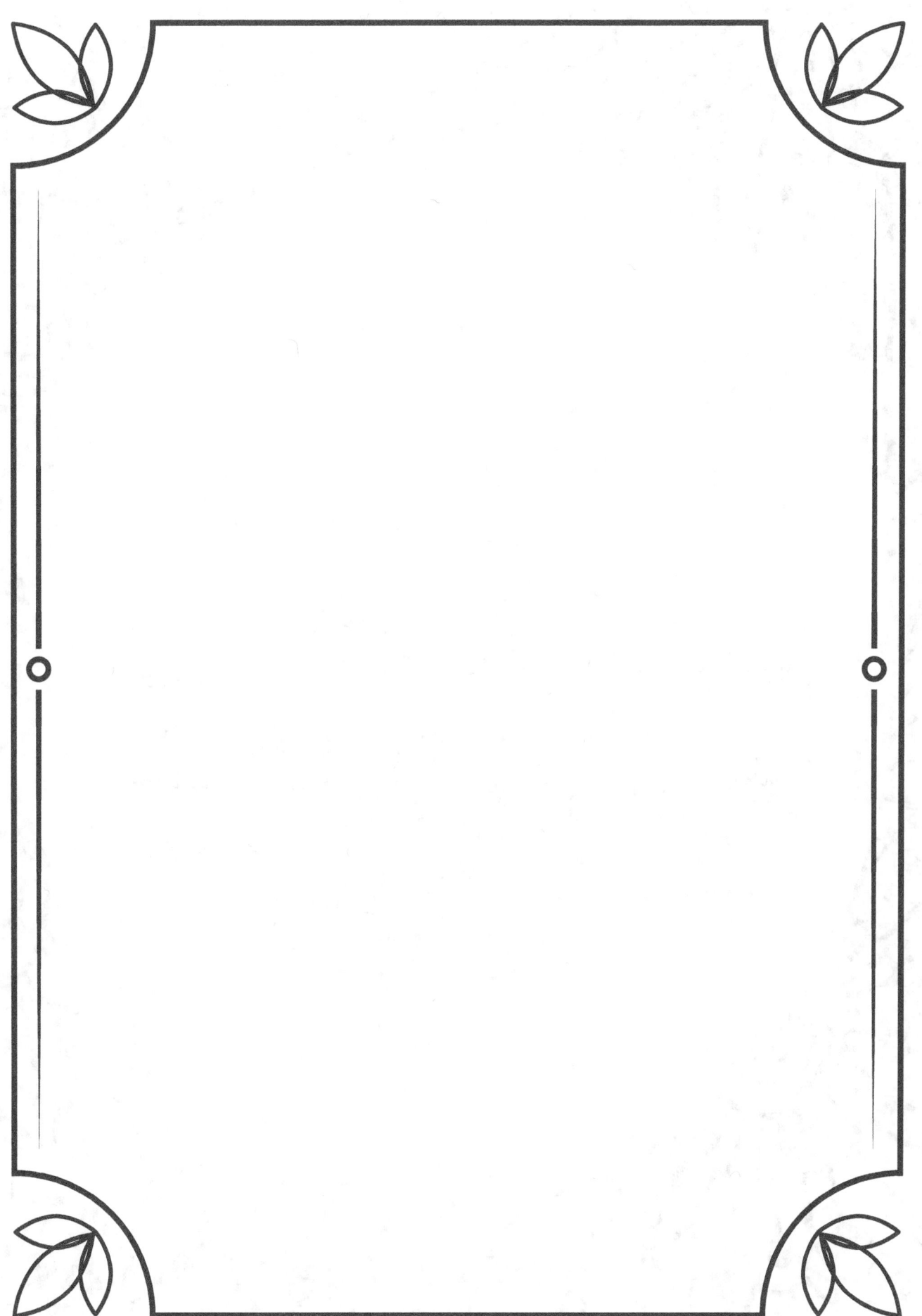

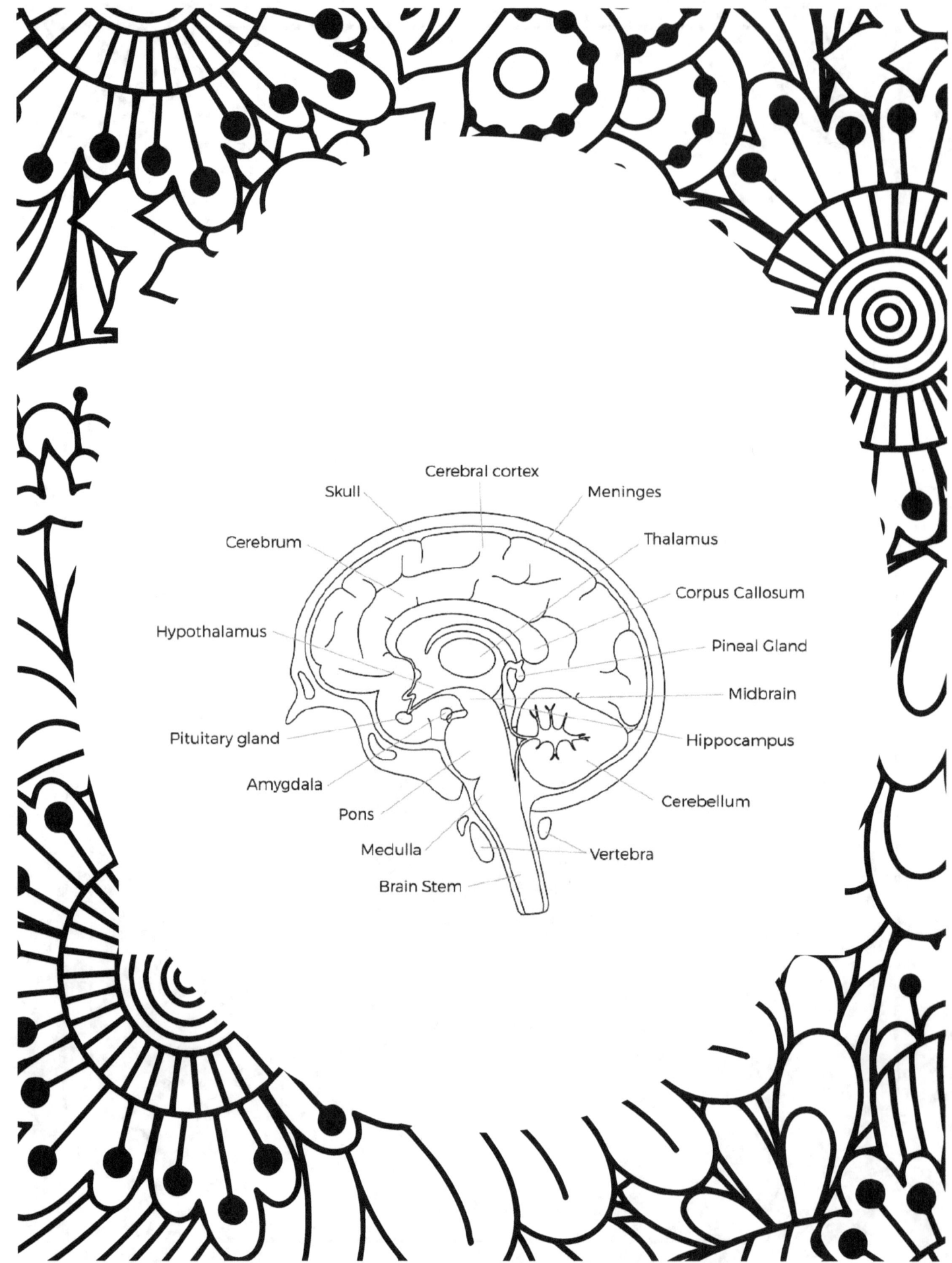

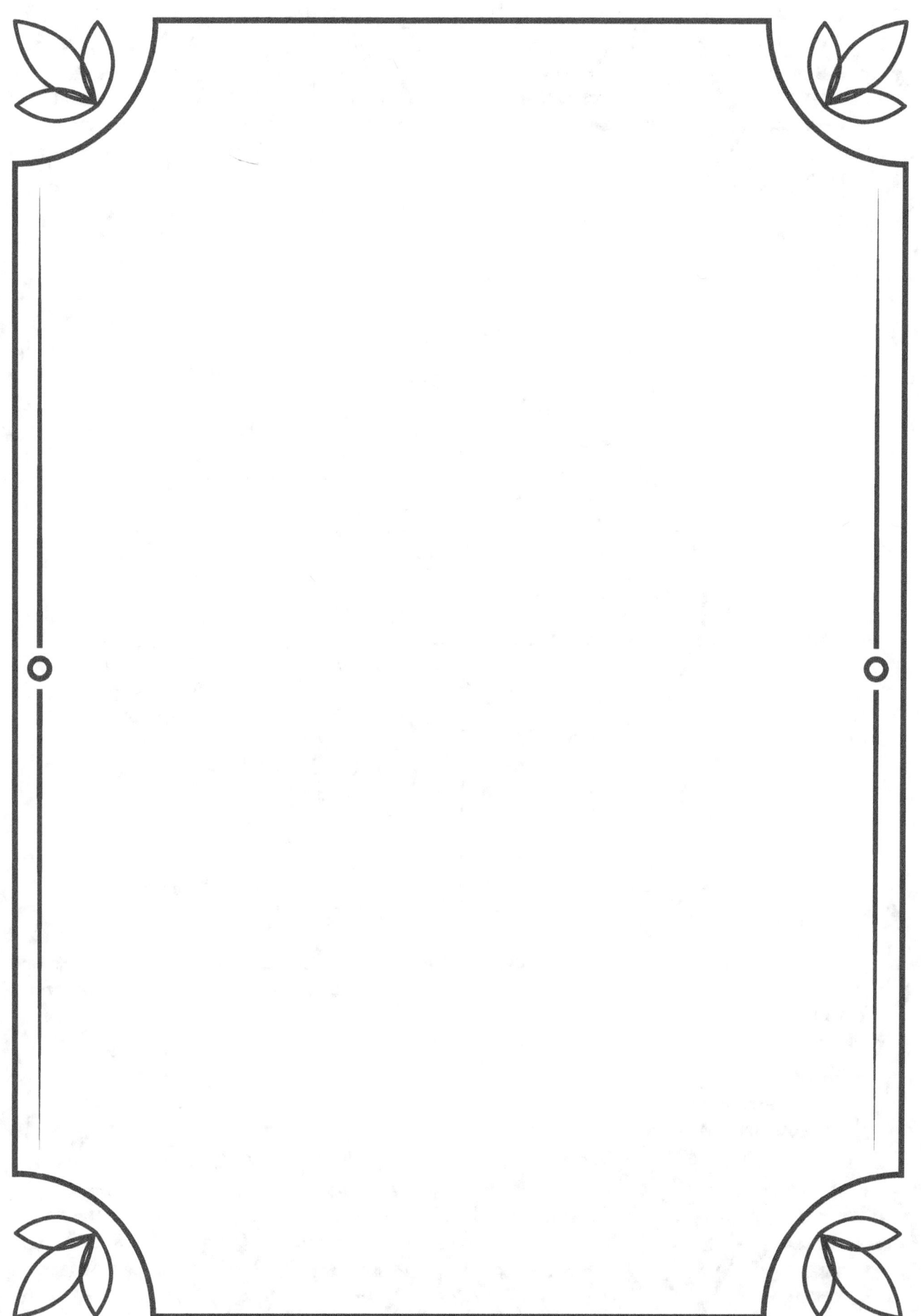

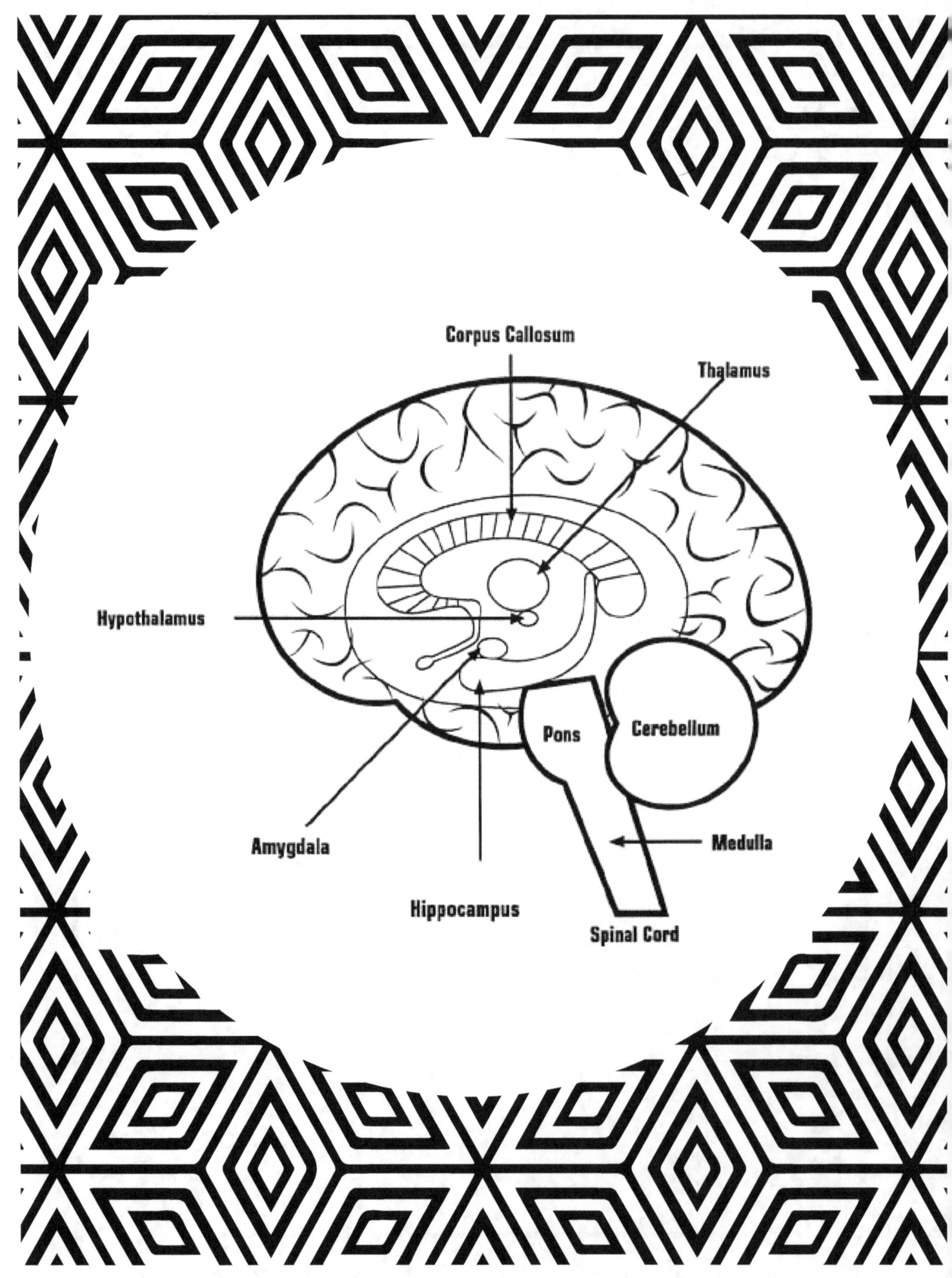

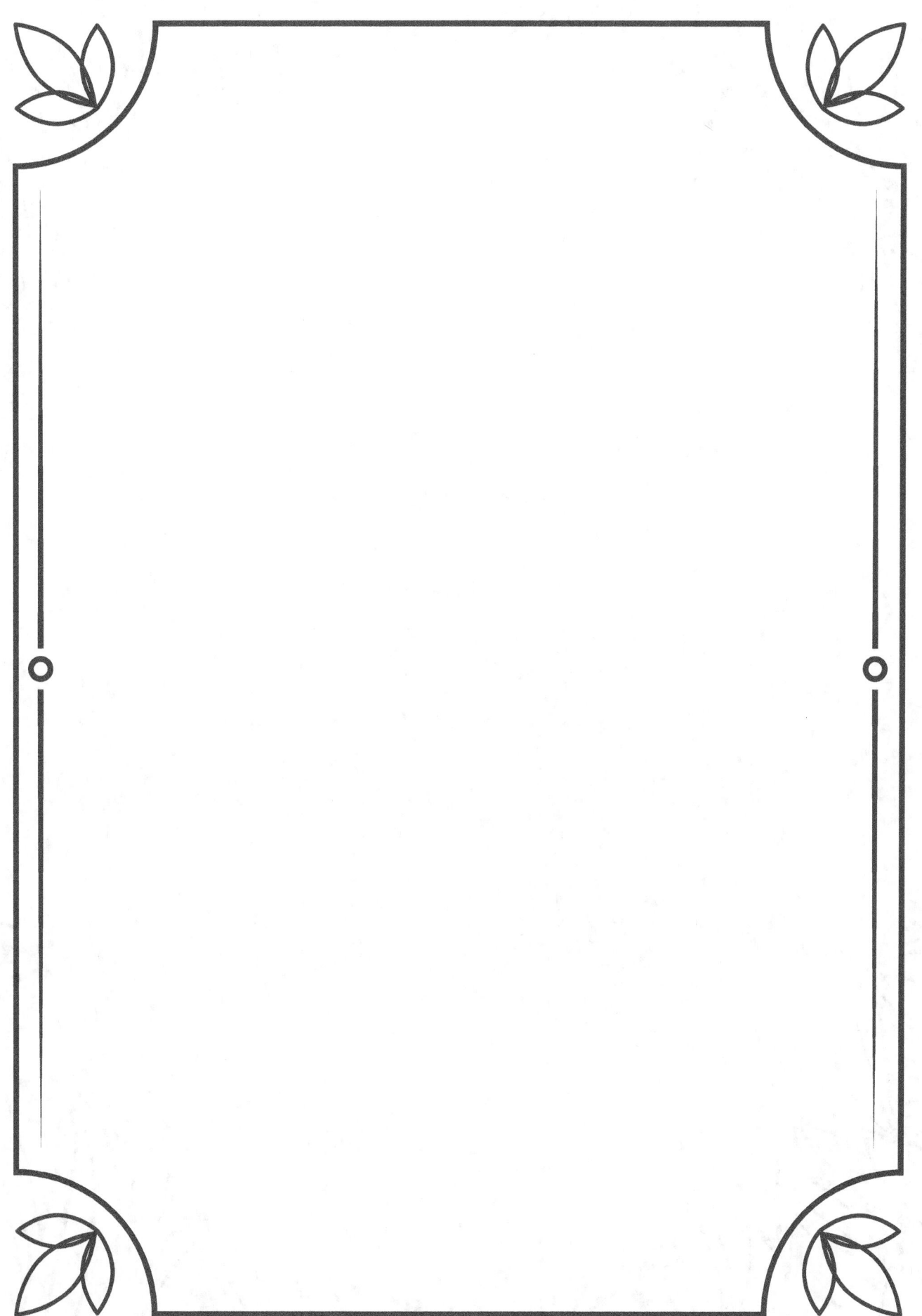

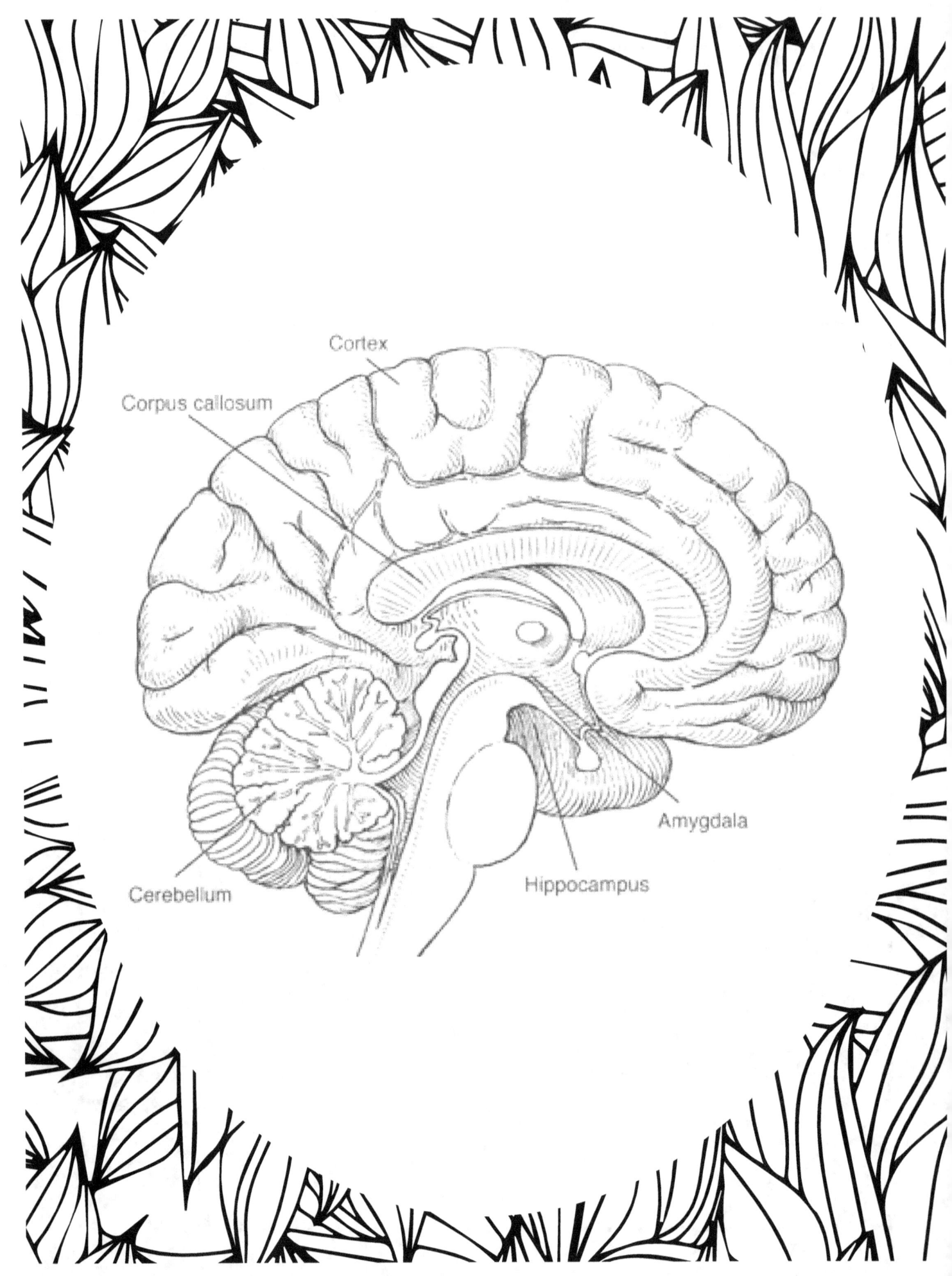

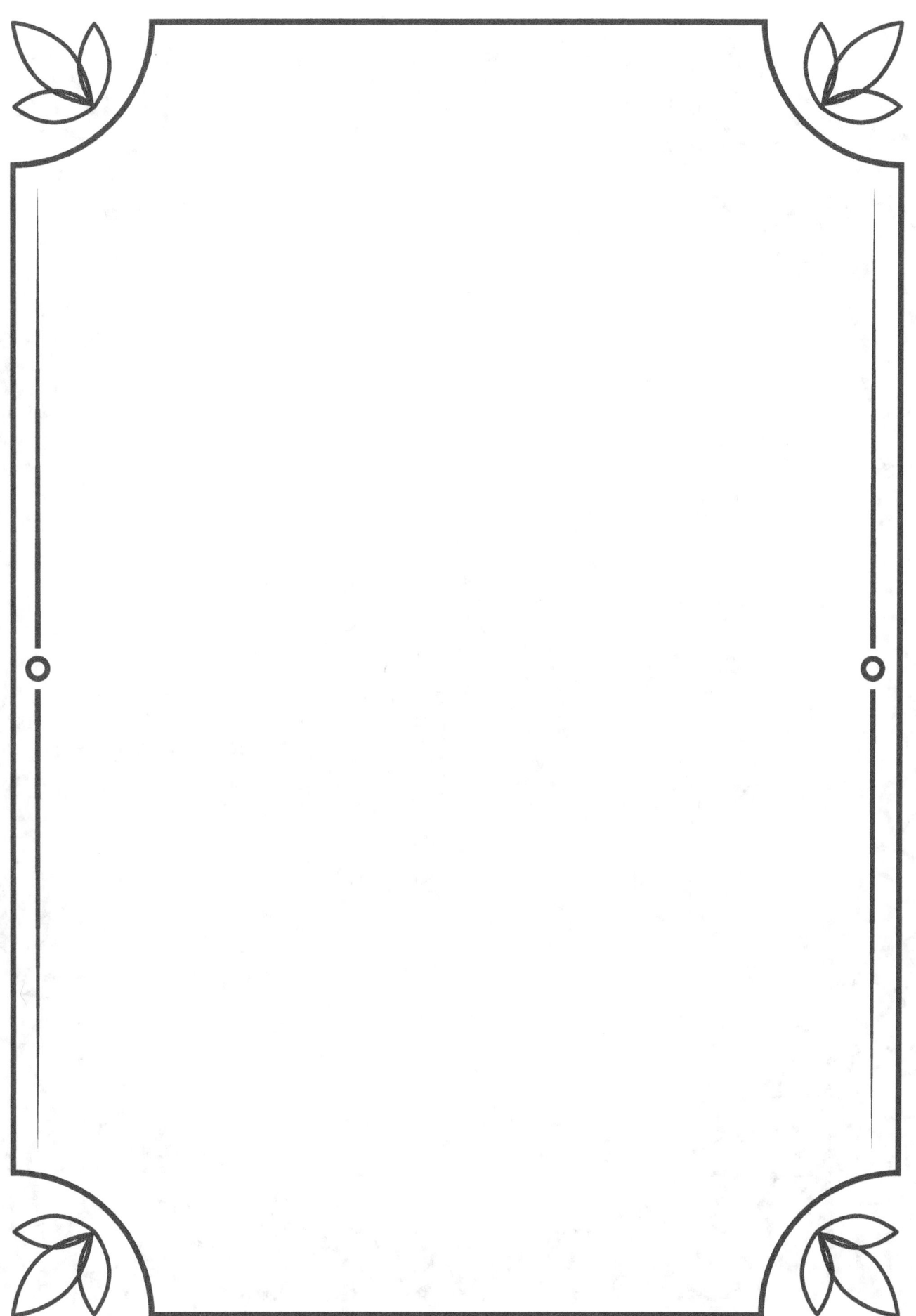

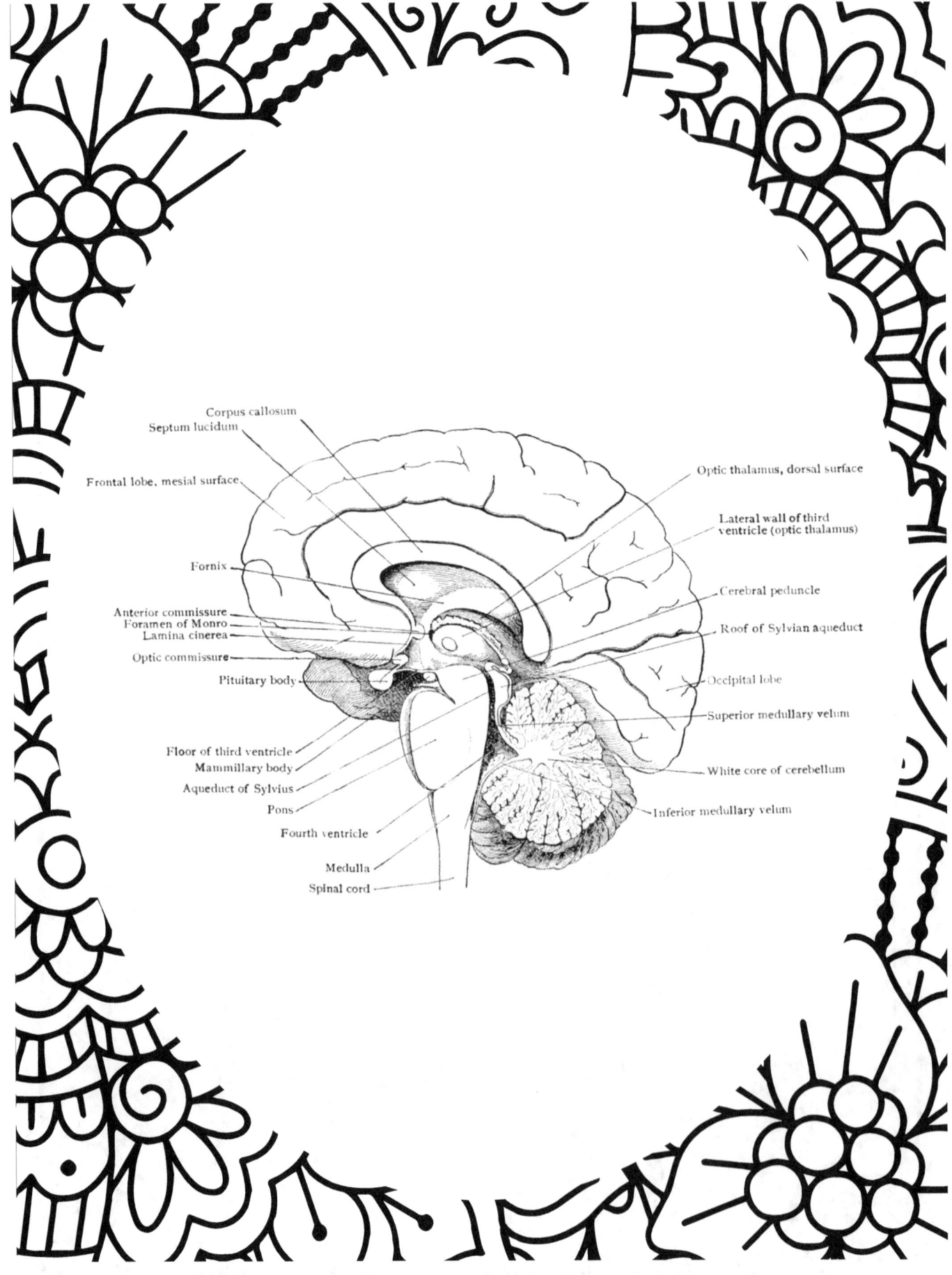

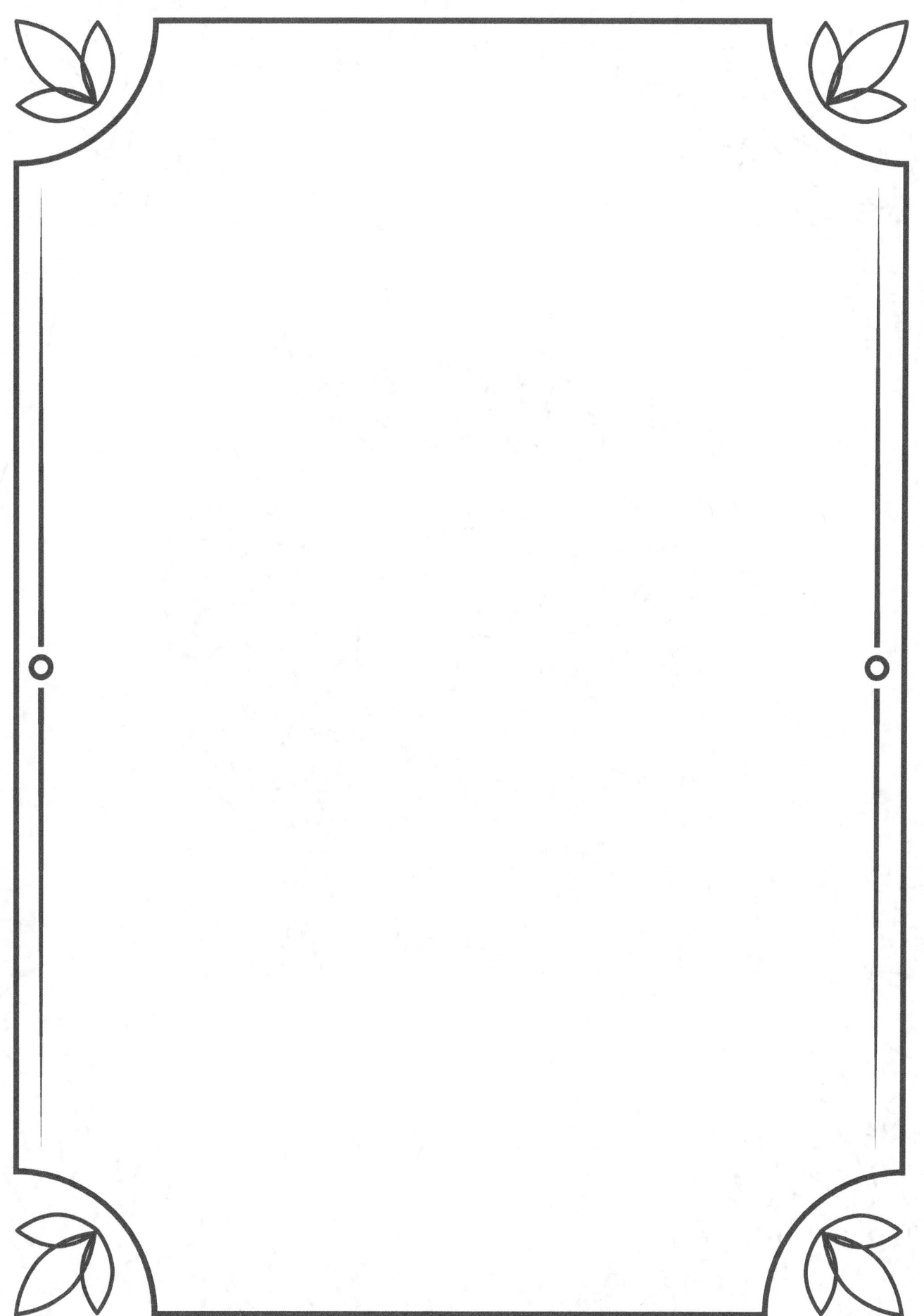

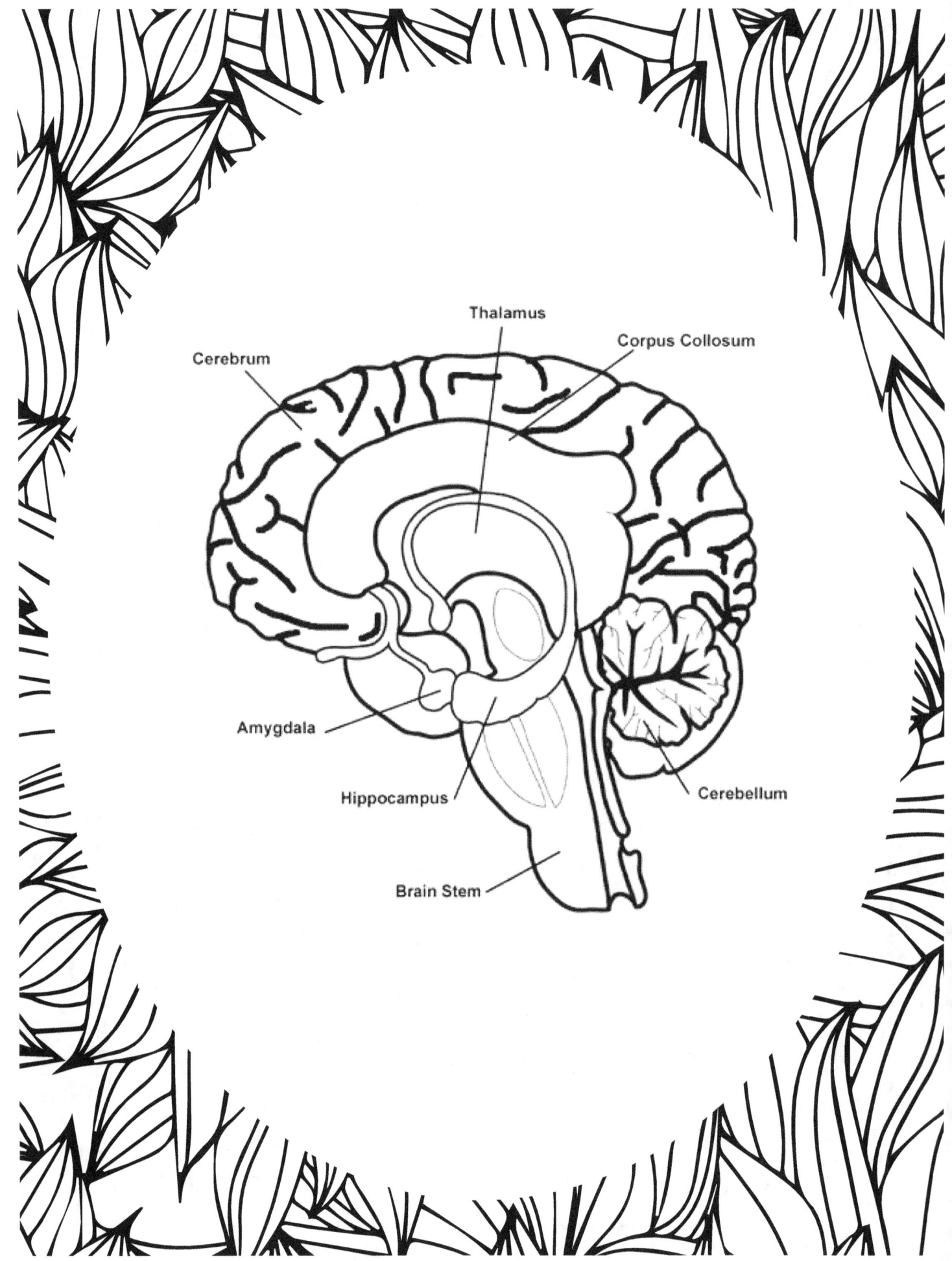

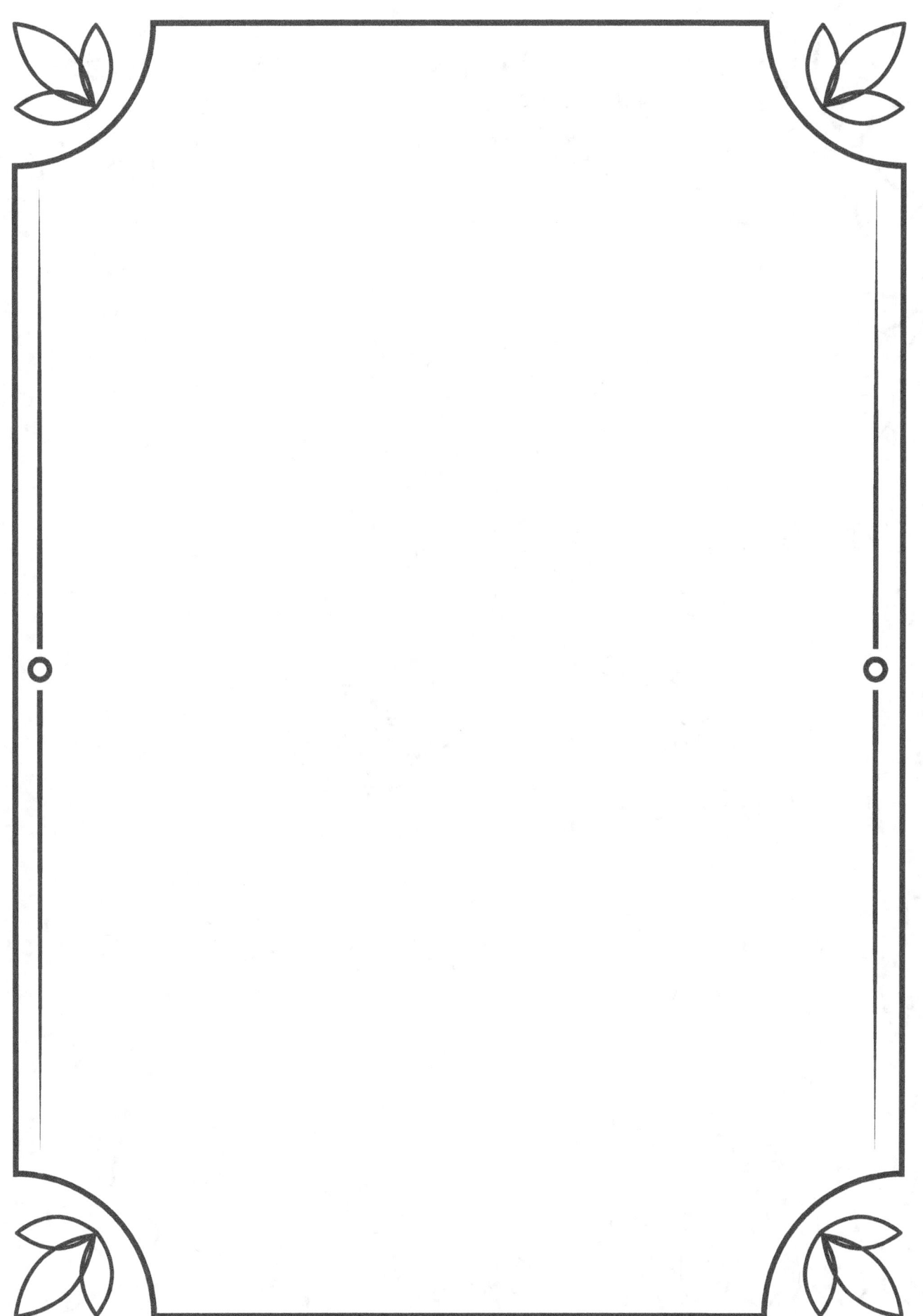

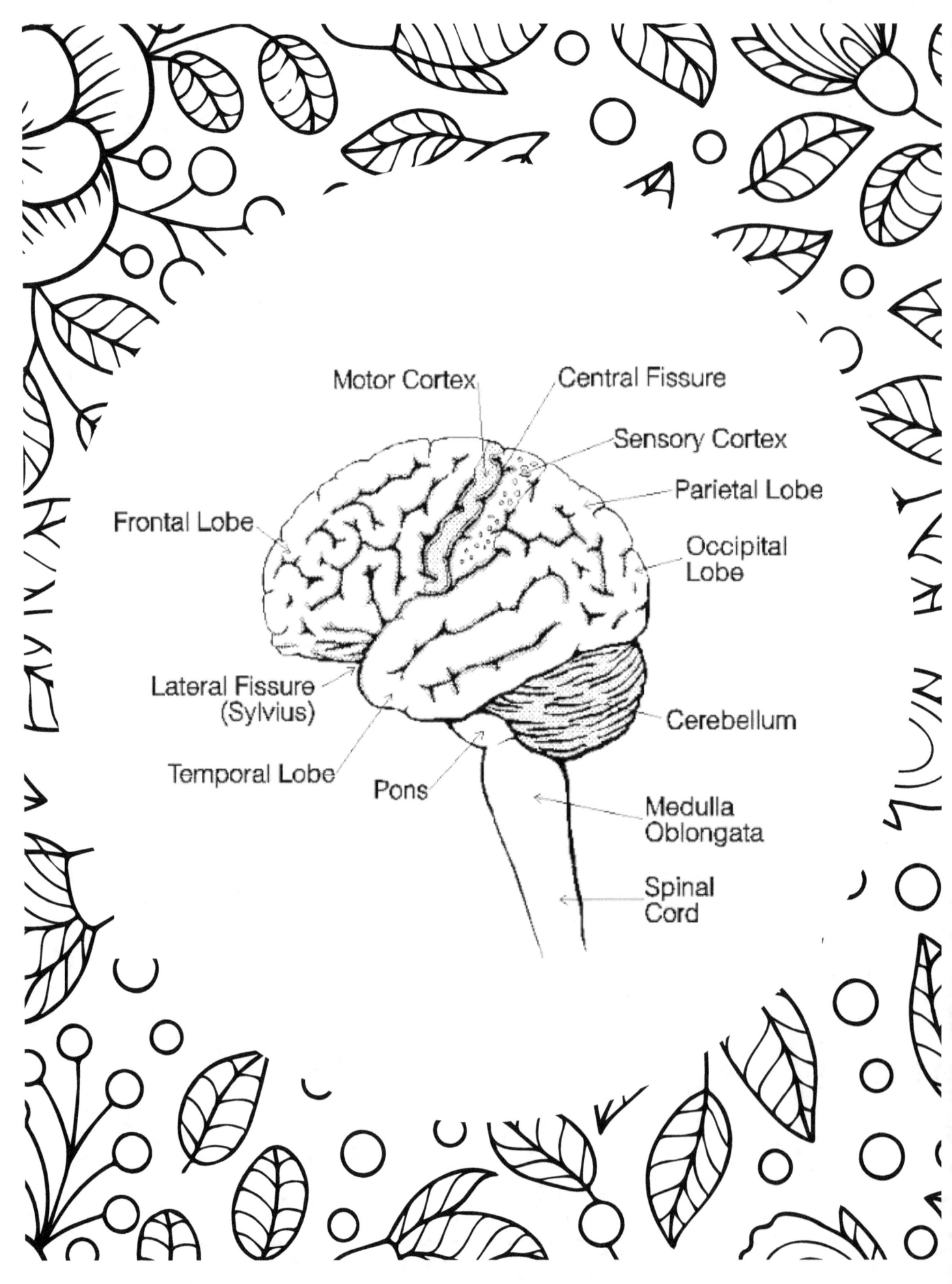

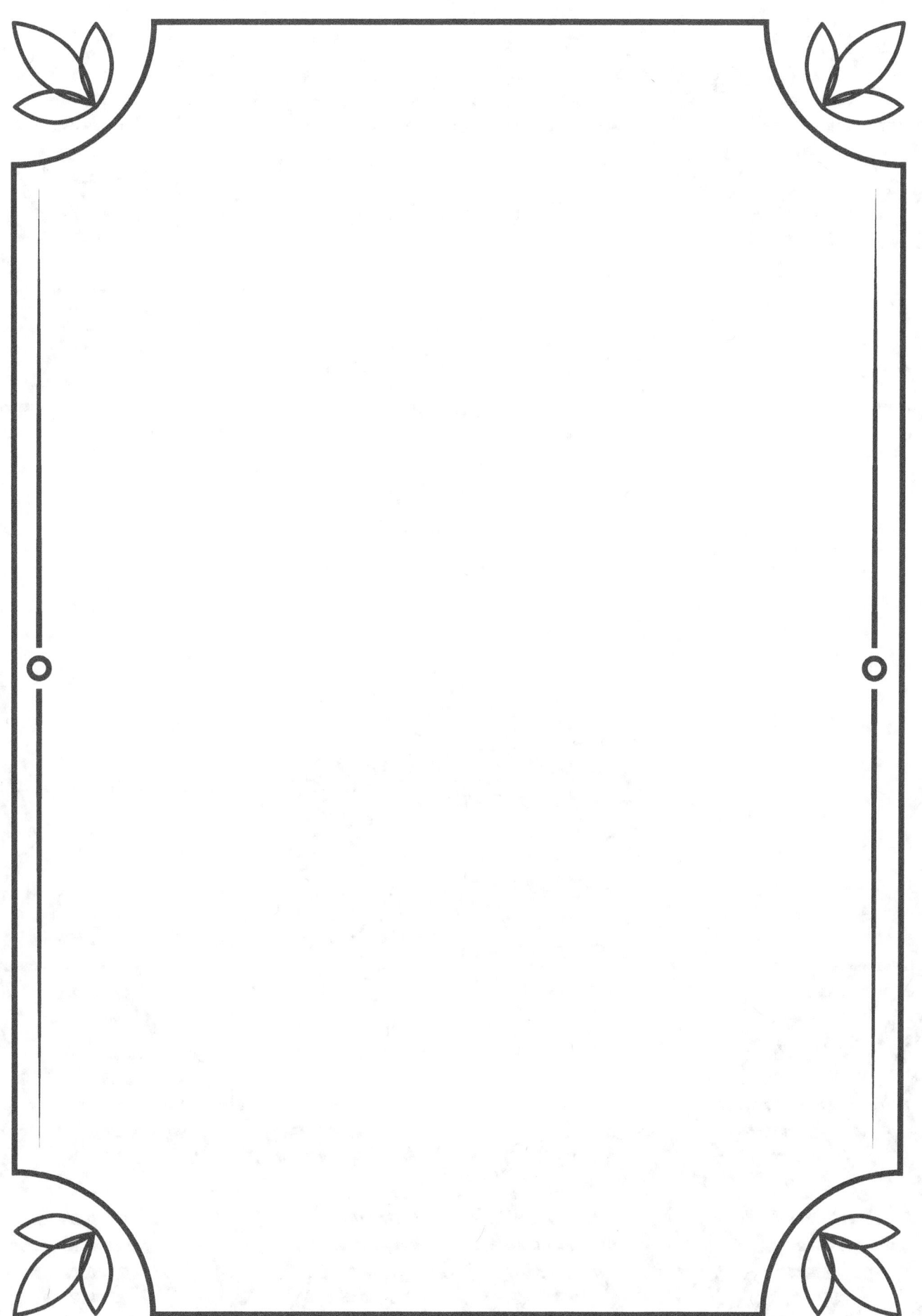

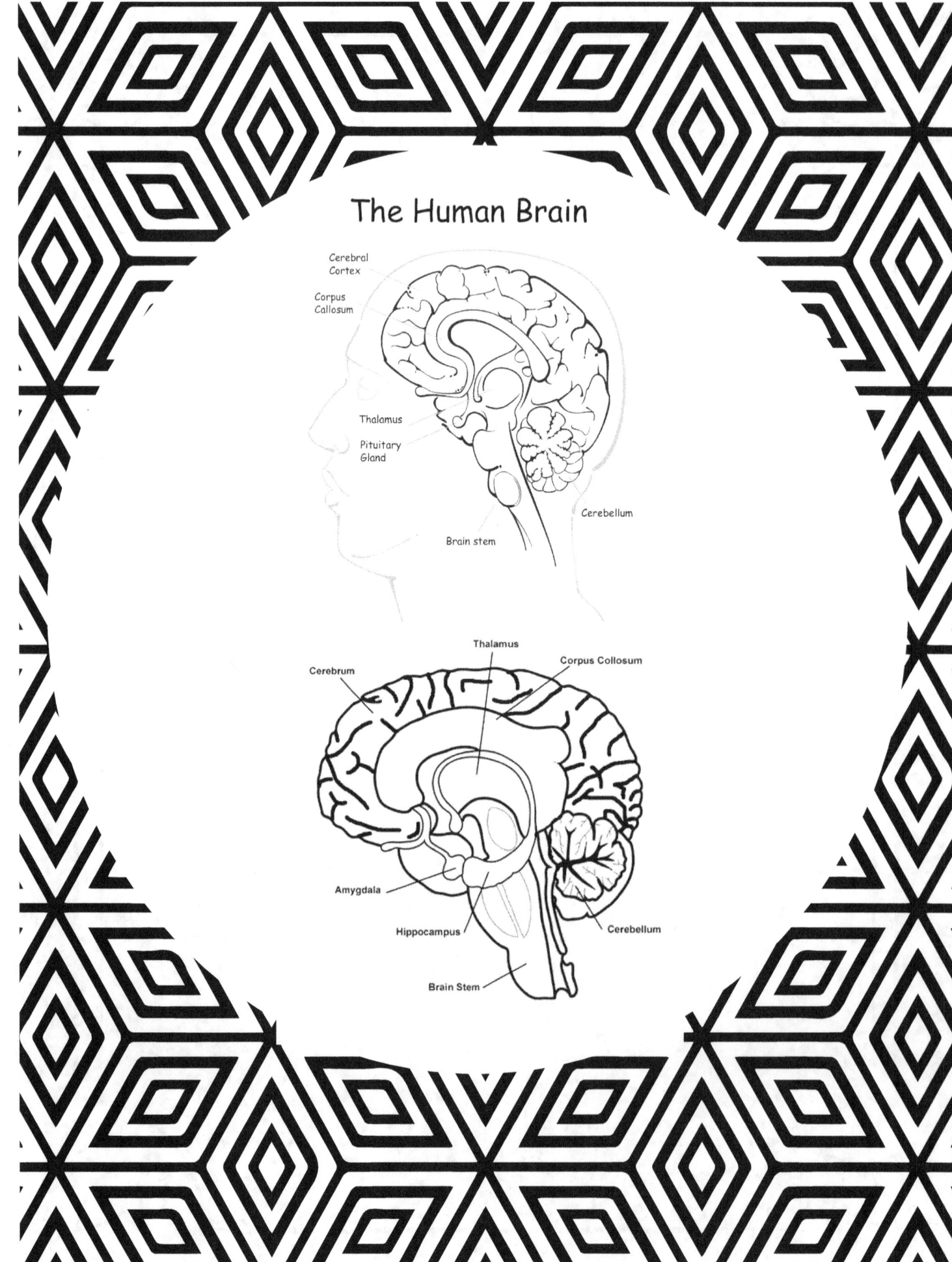

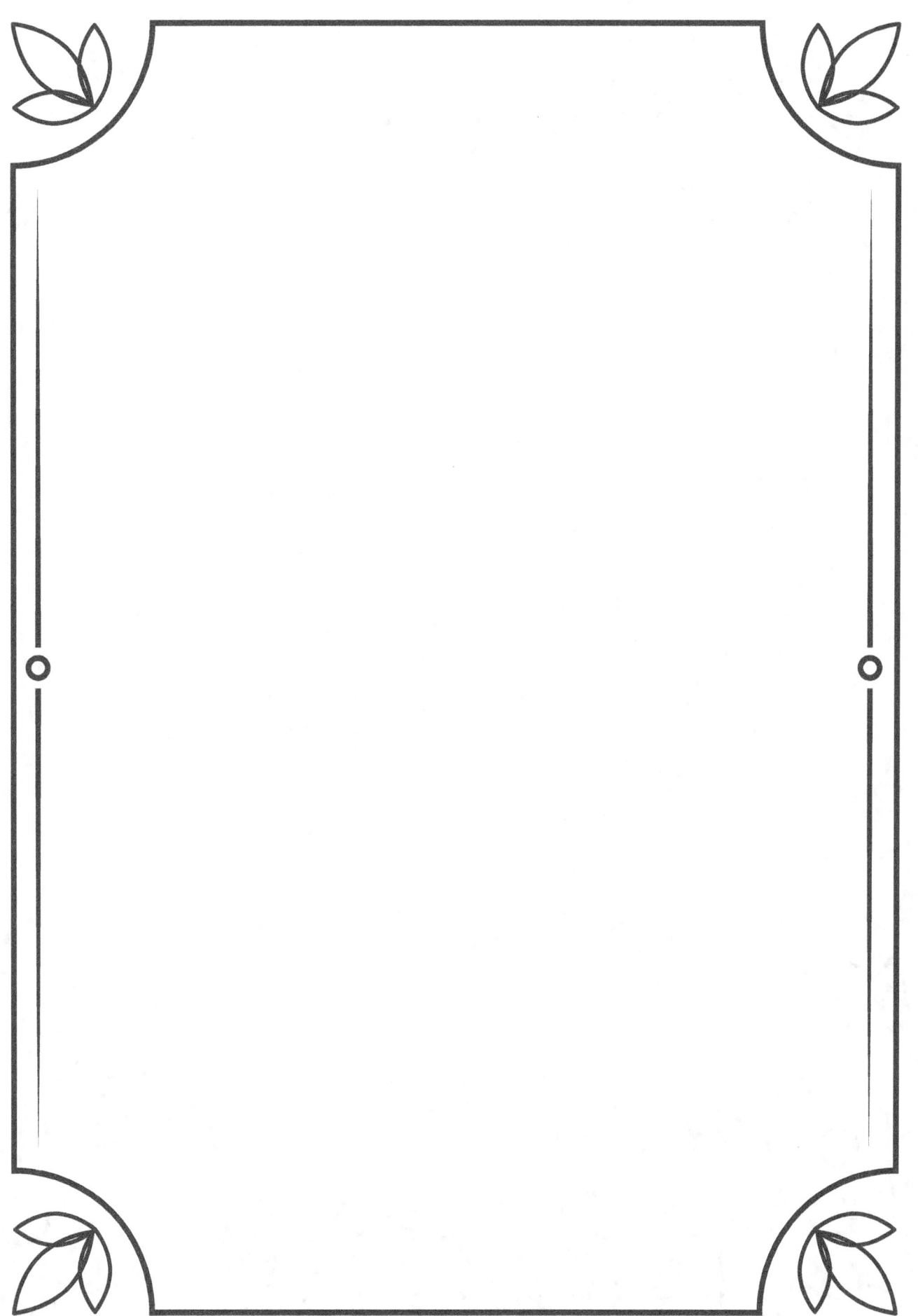

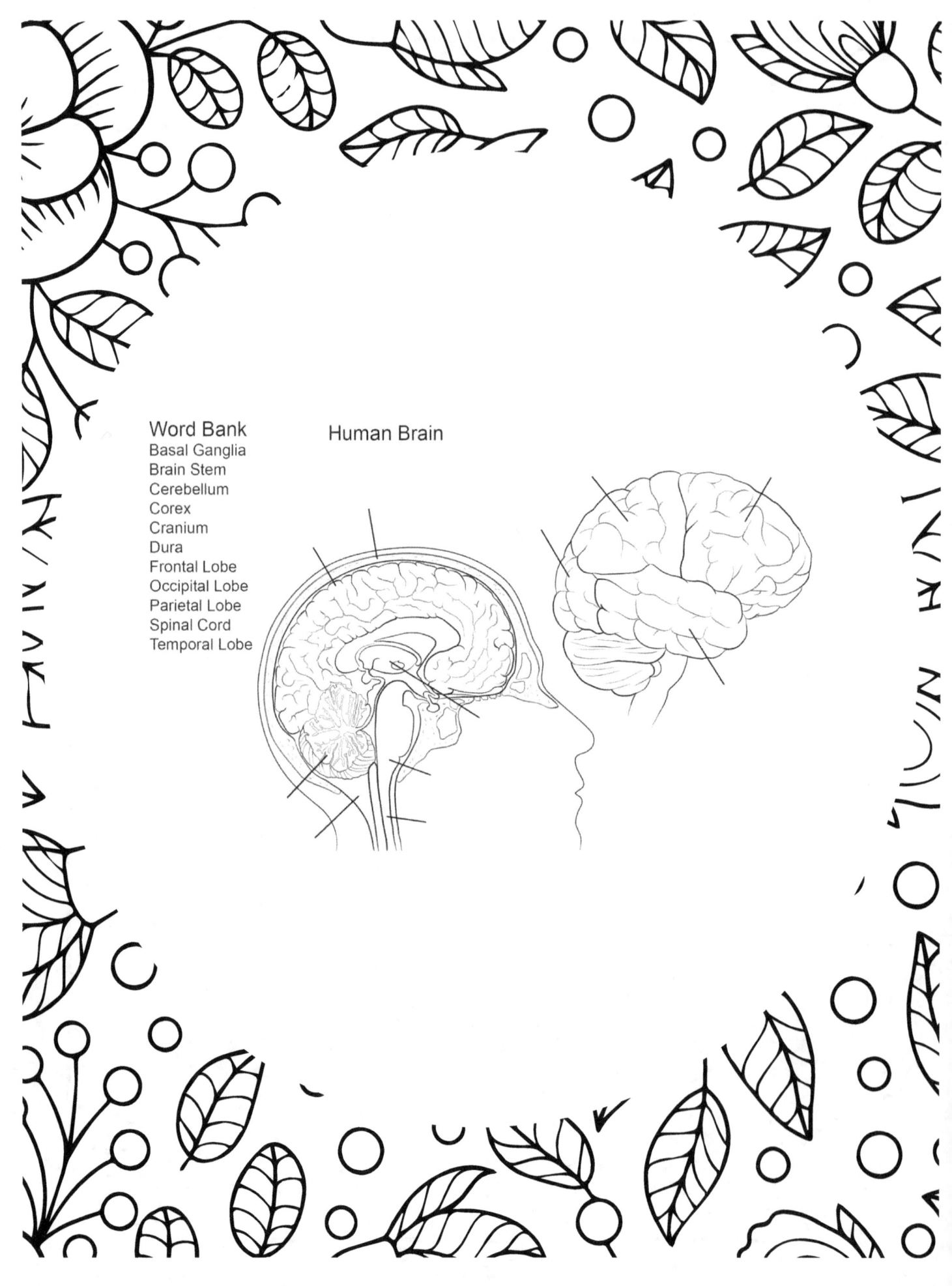

Word Bank
Basal Ganglia
Brain Stem
Cerebellum
Corex
Cranium
Dura
Frontal Lobe
Occipital Lobe
Parietal Lobe
Spinal Cord
Temporal Lobe

Human Brain

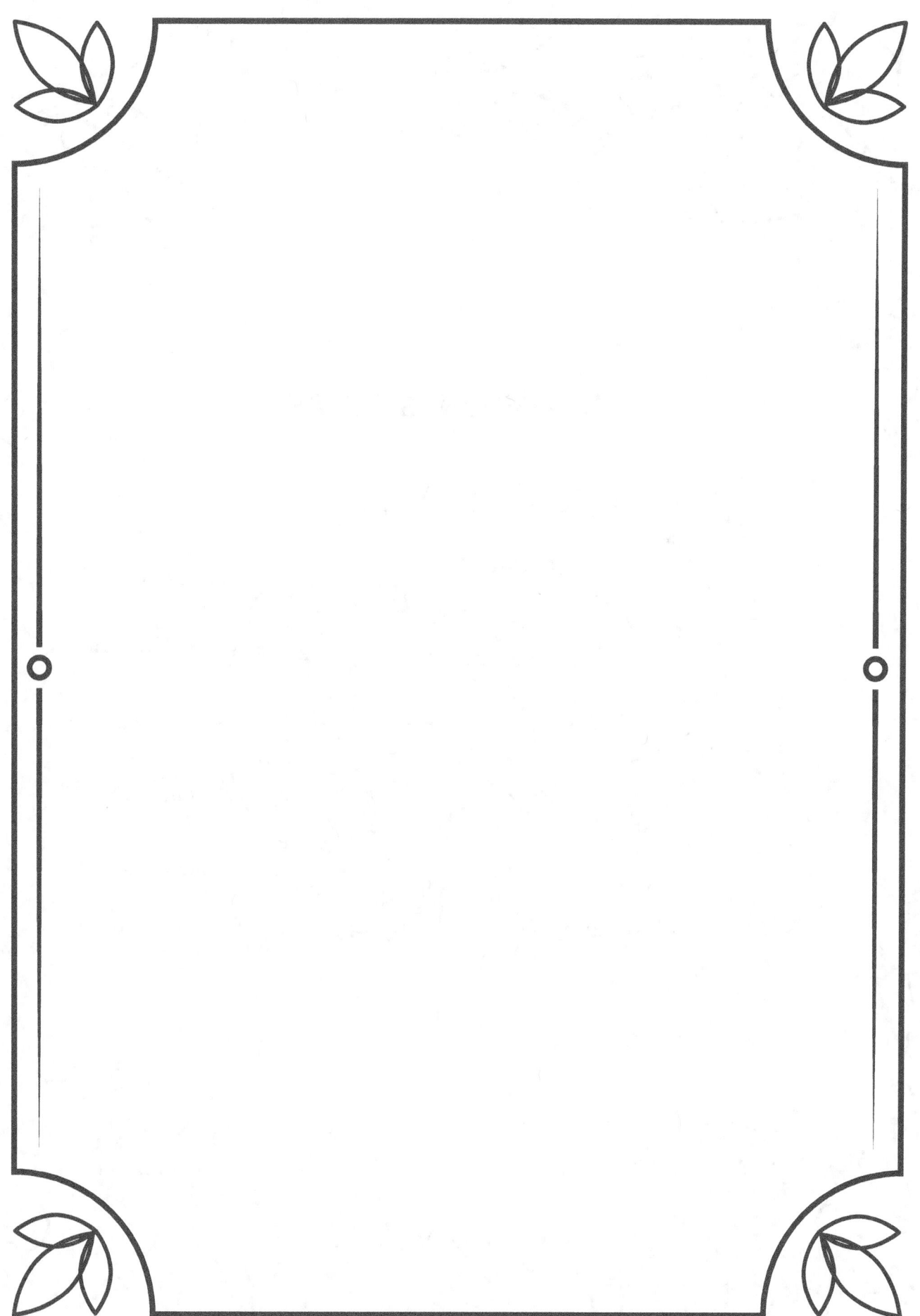

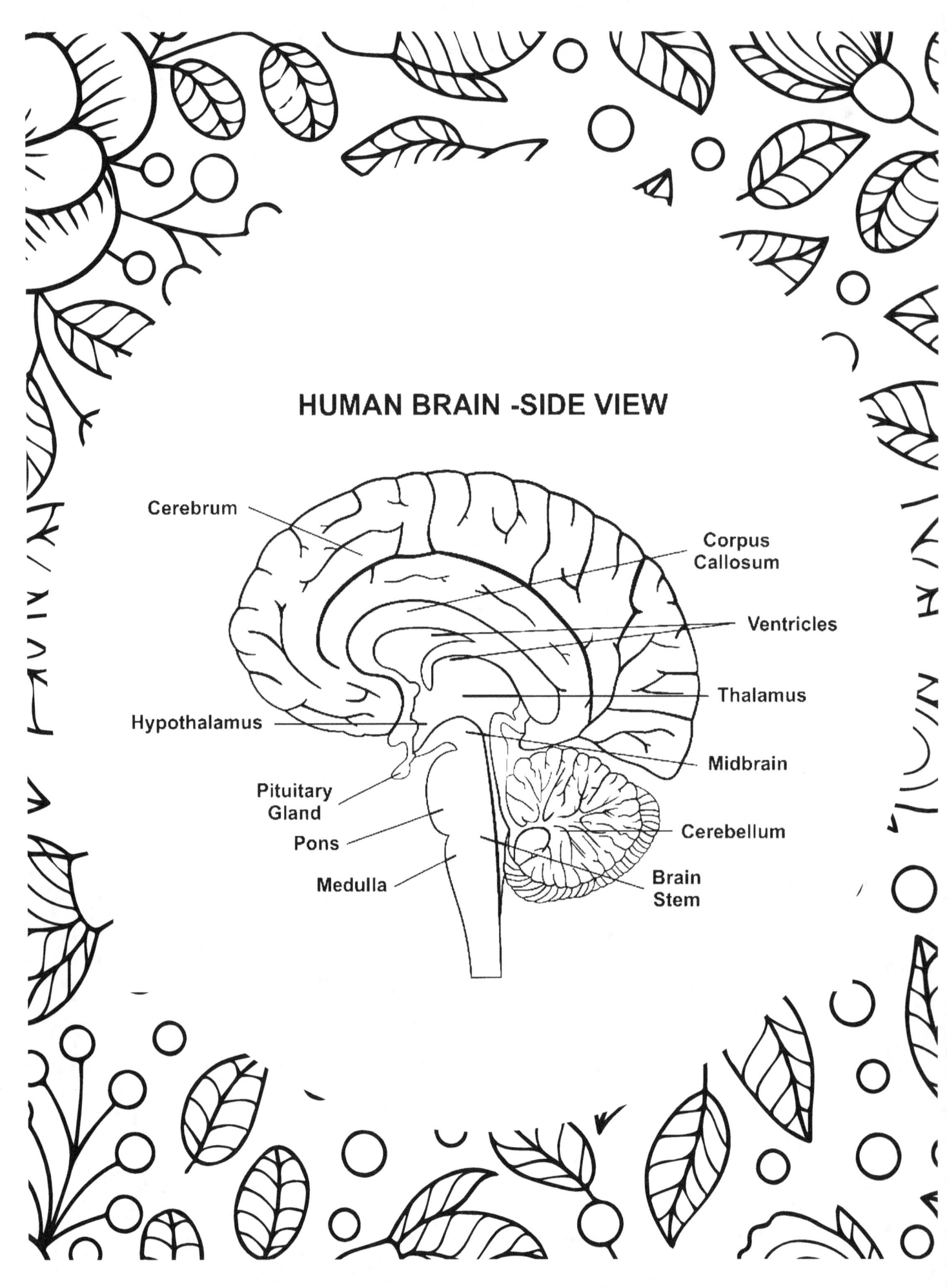

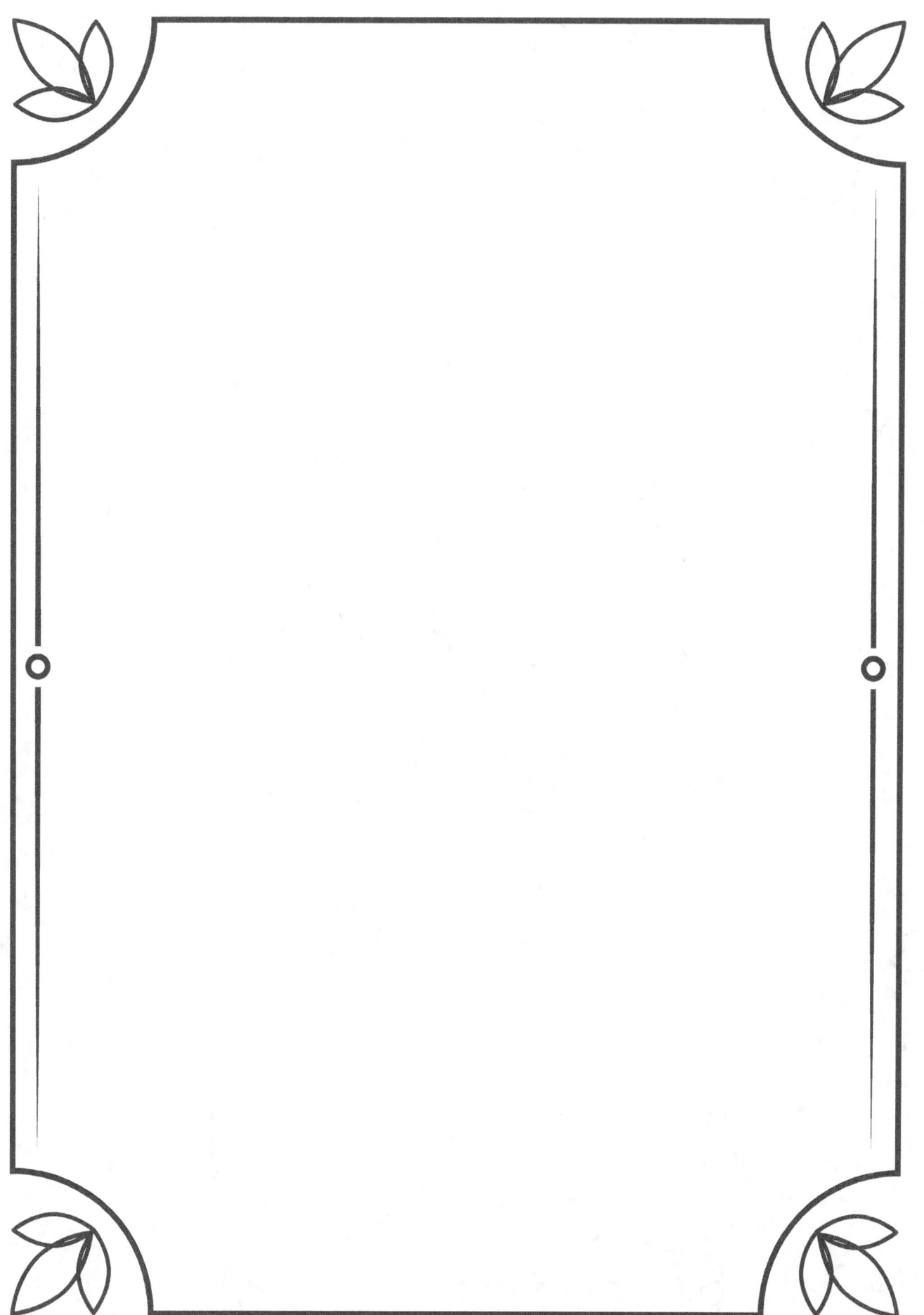

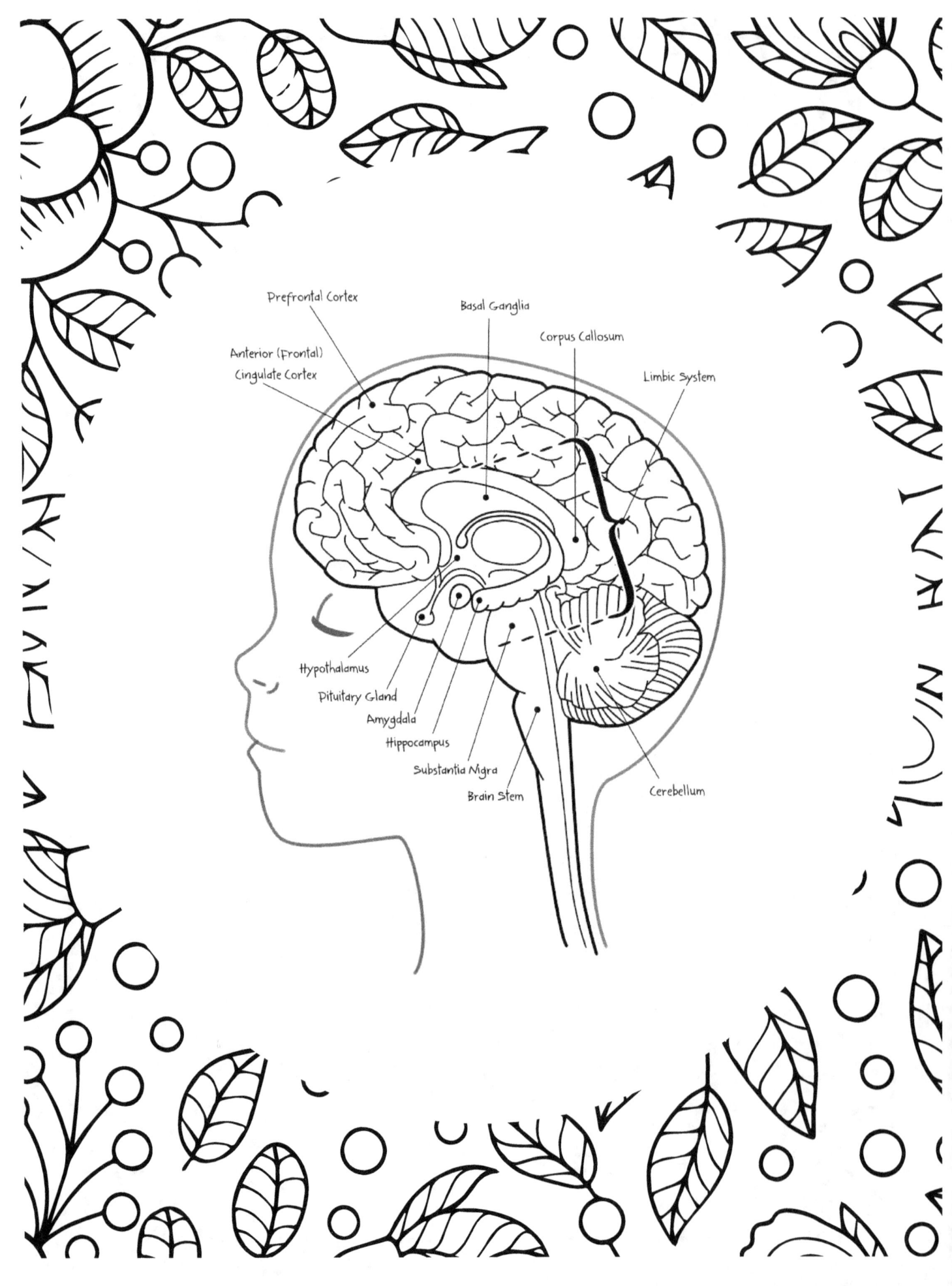

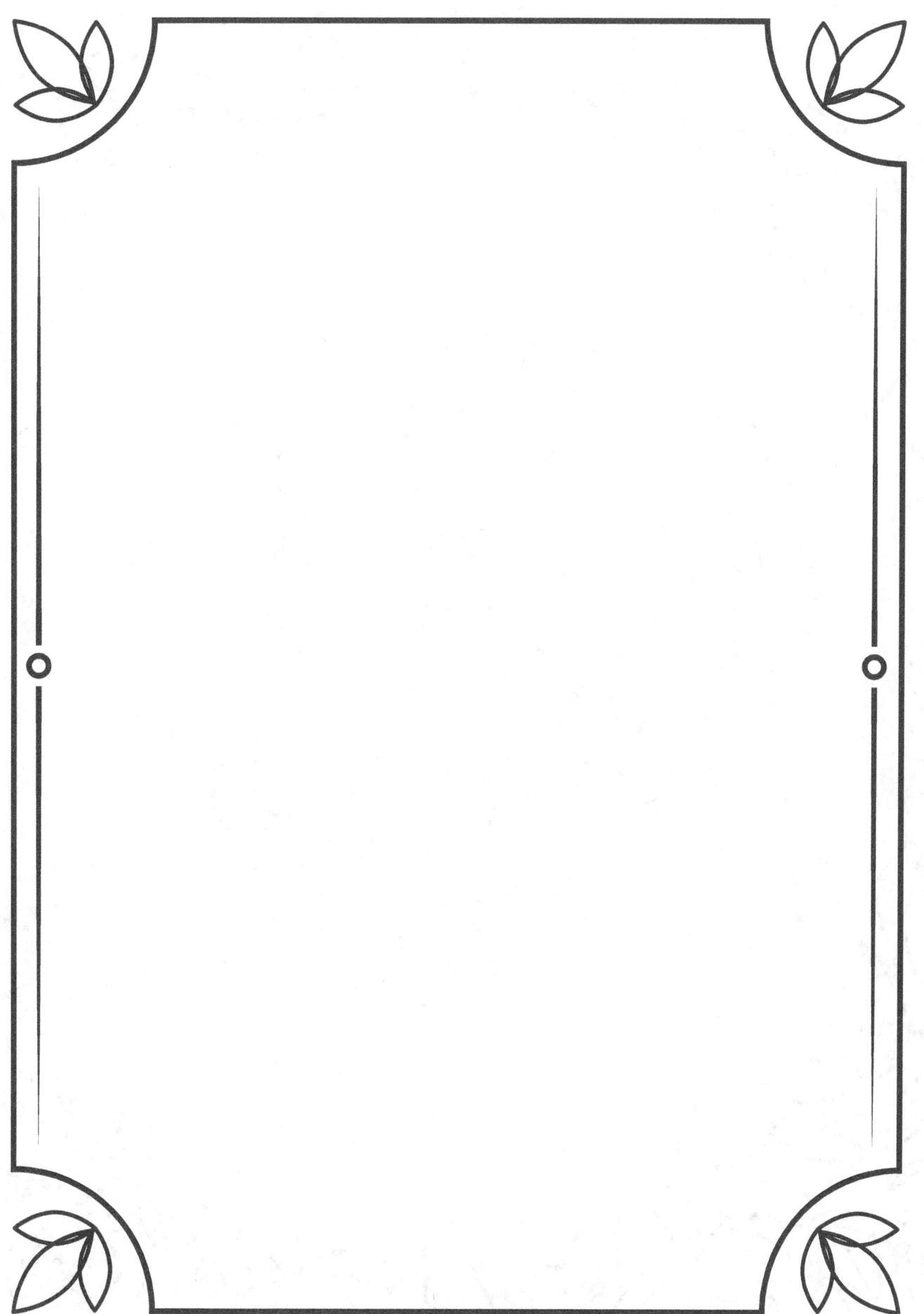

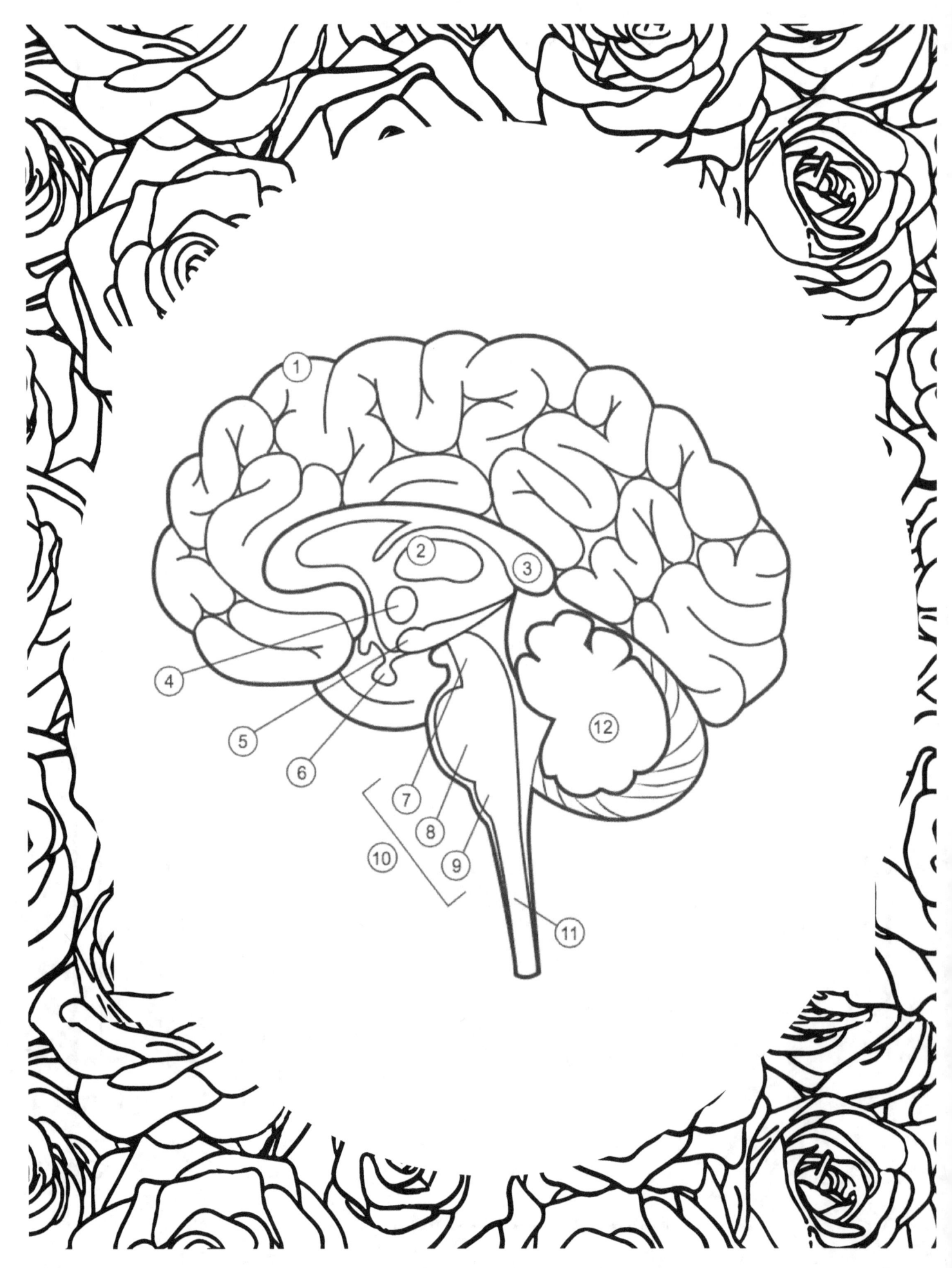

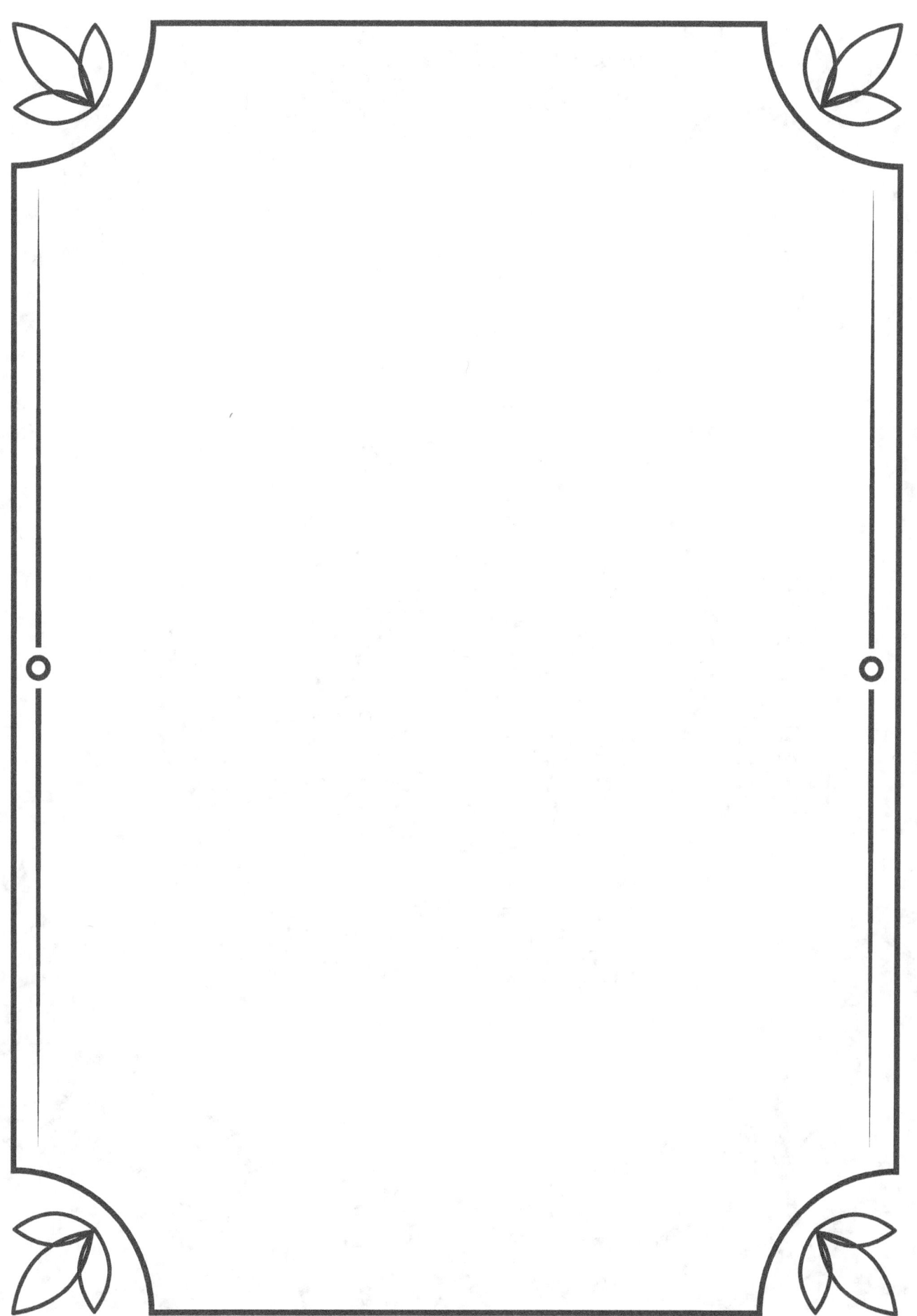

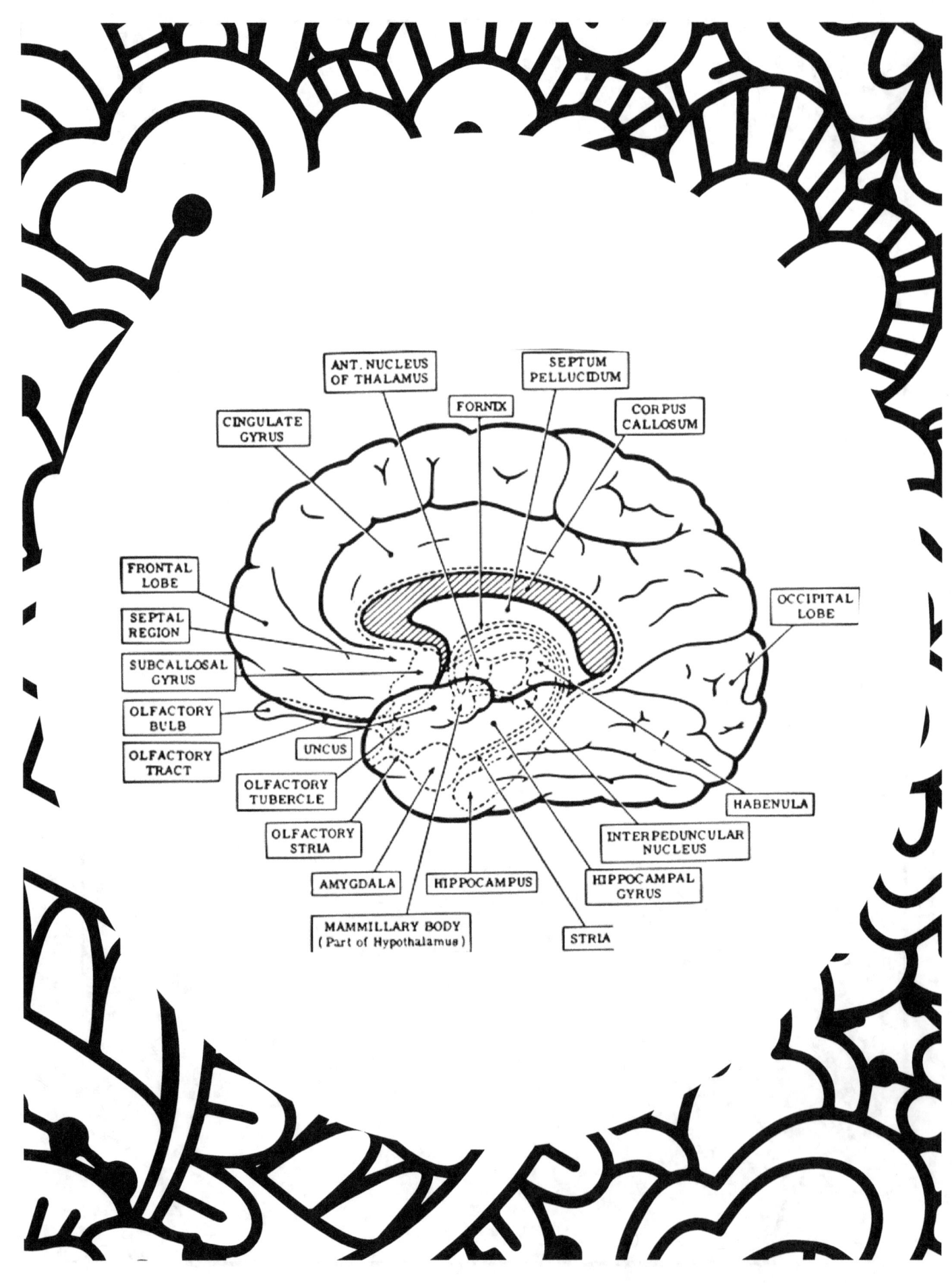

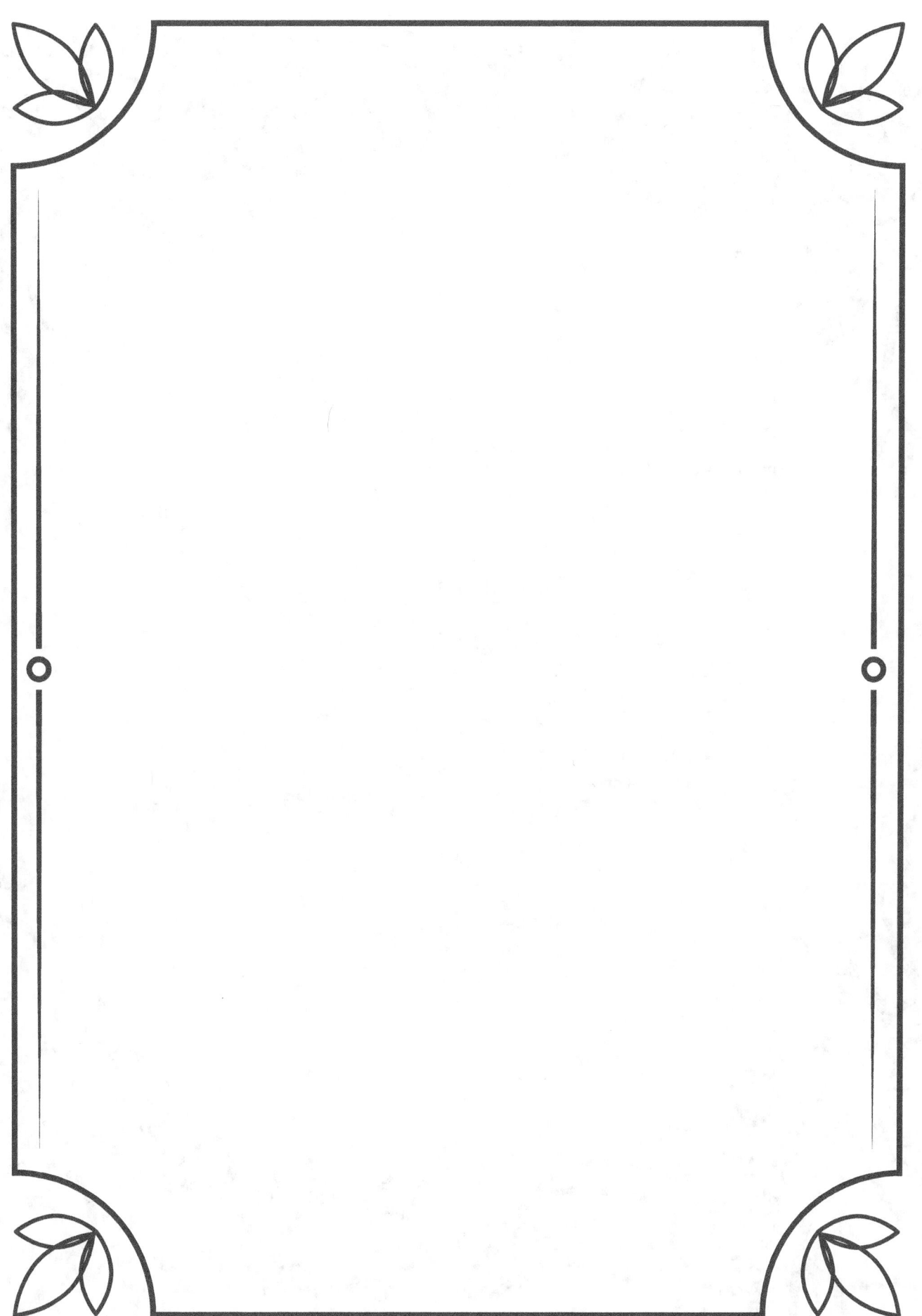

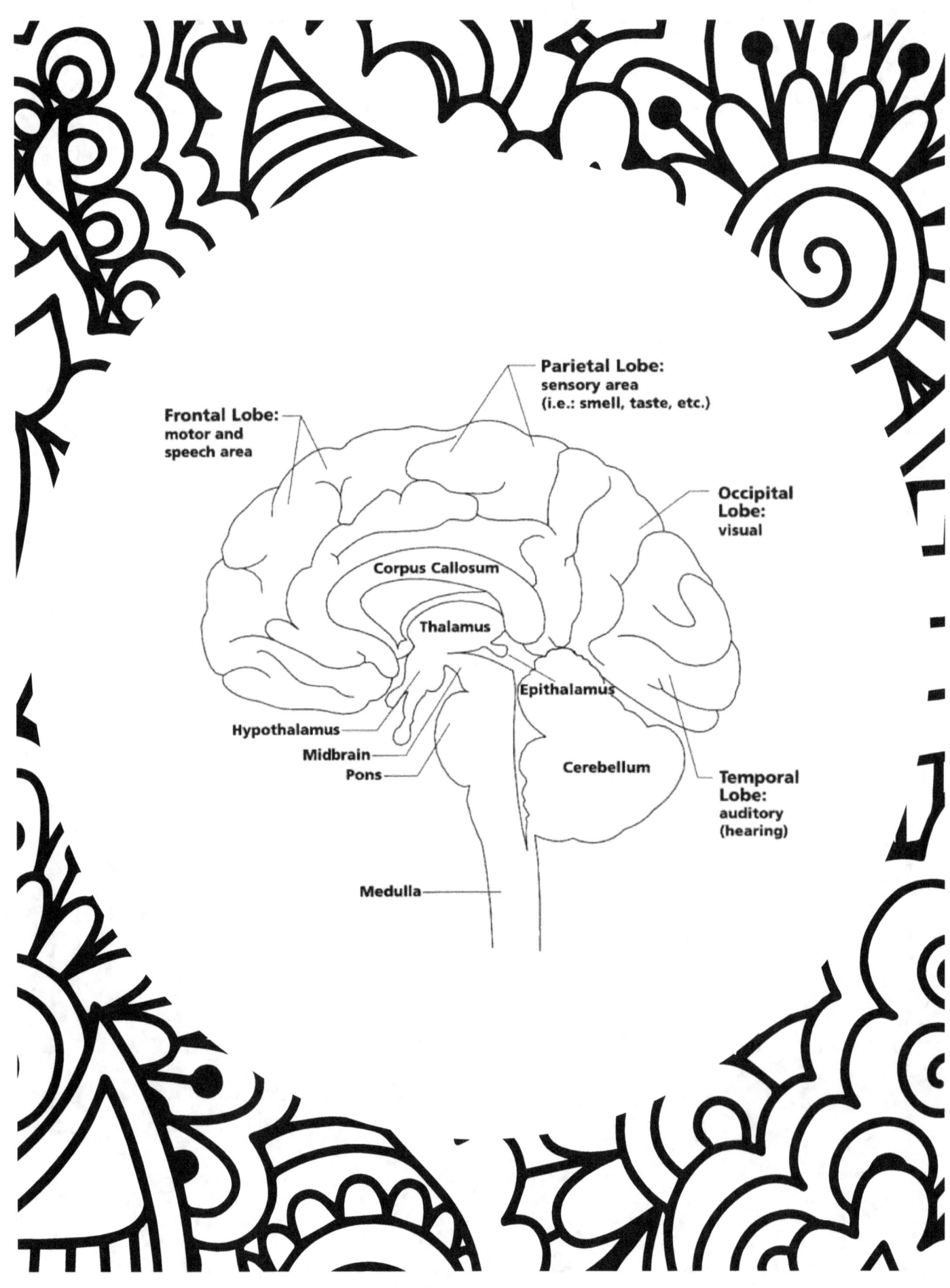

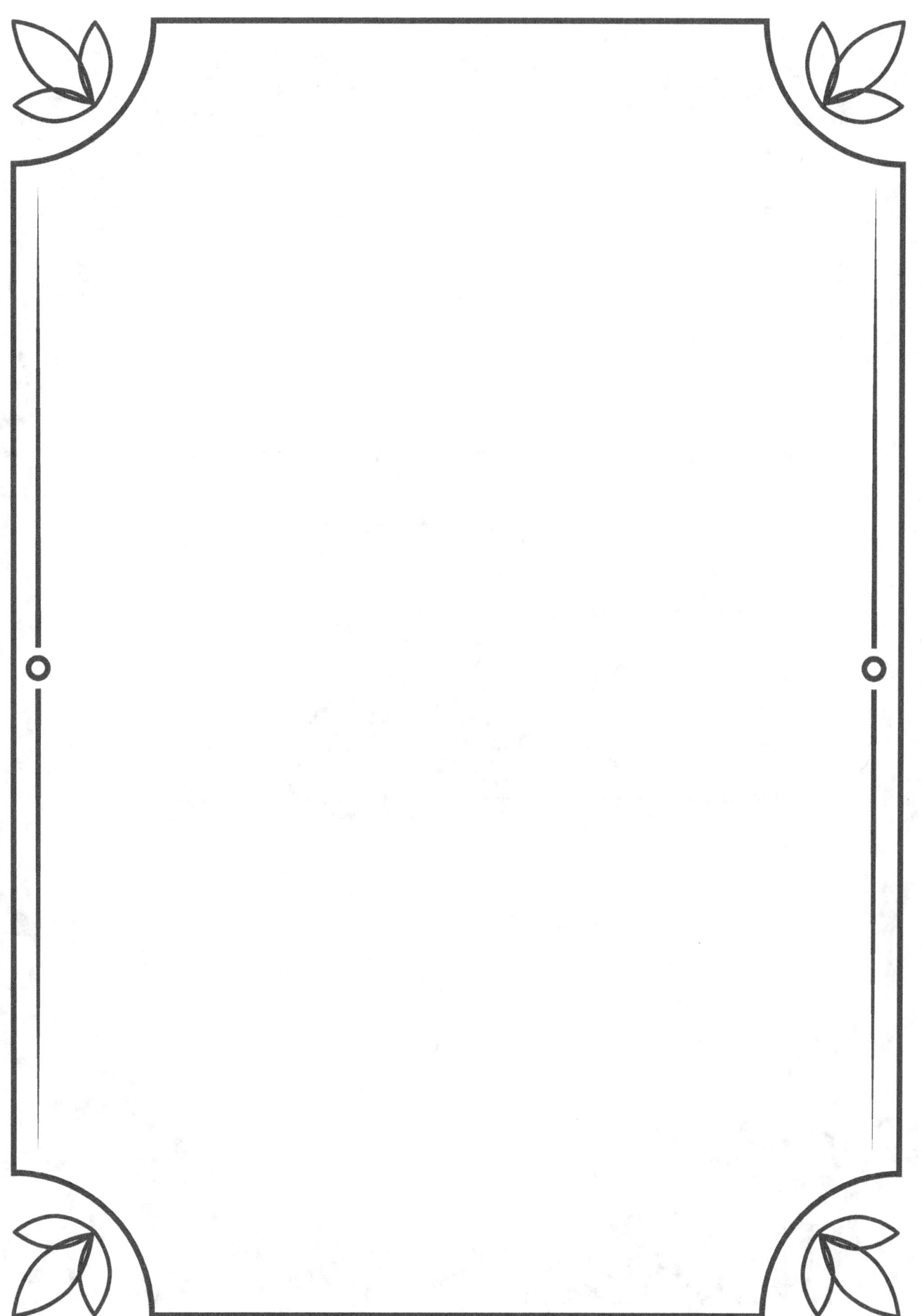

The Major Portions of the Brain Include the Cerebrum, Cerebellum and Brain Stem

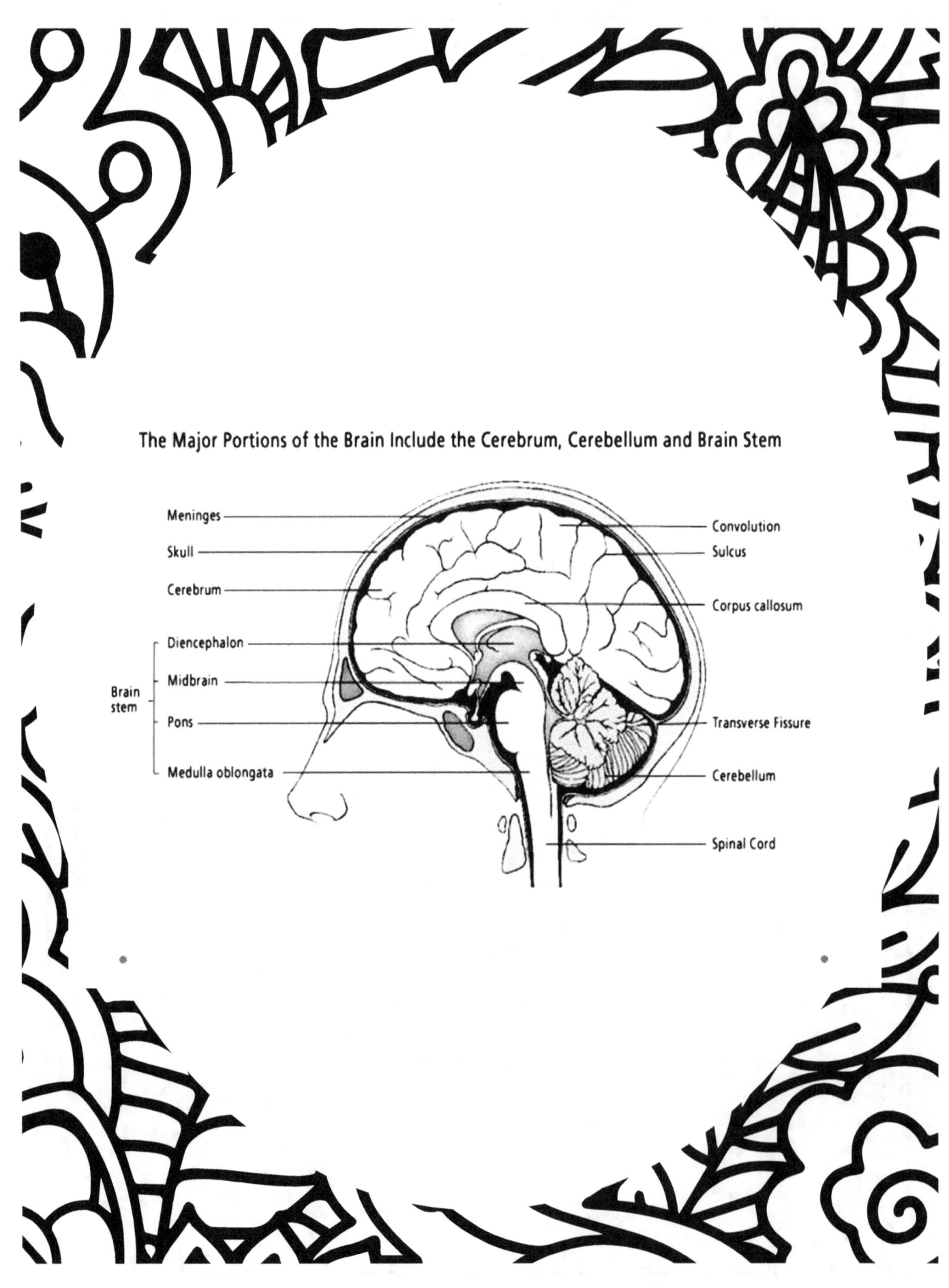

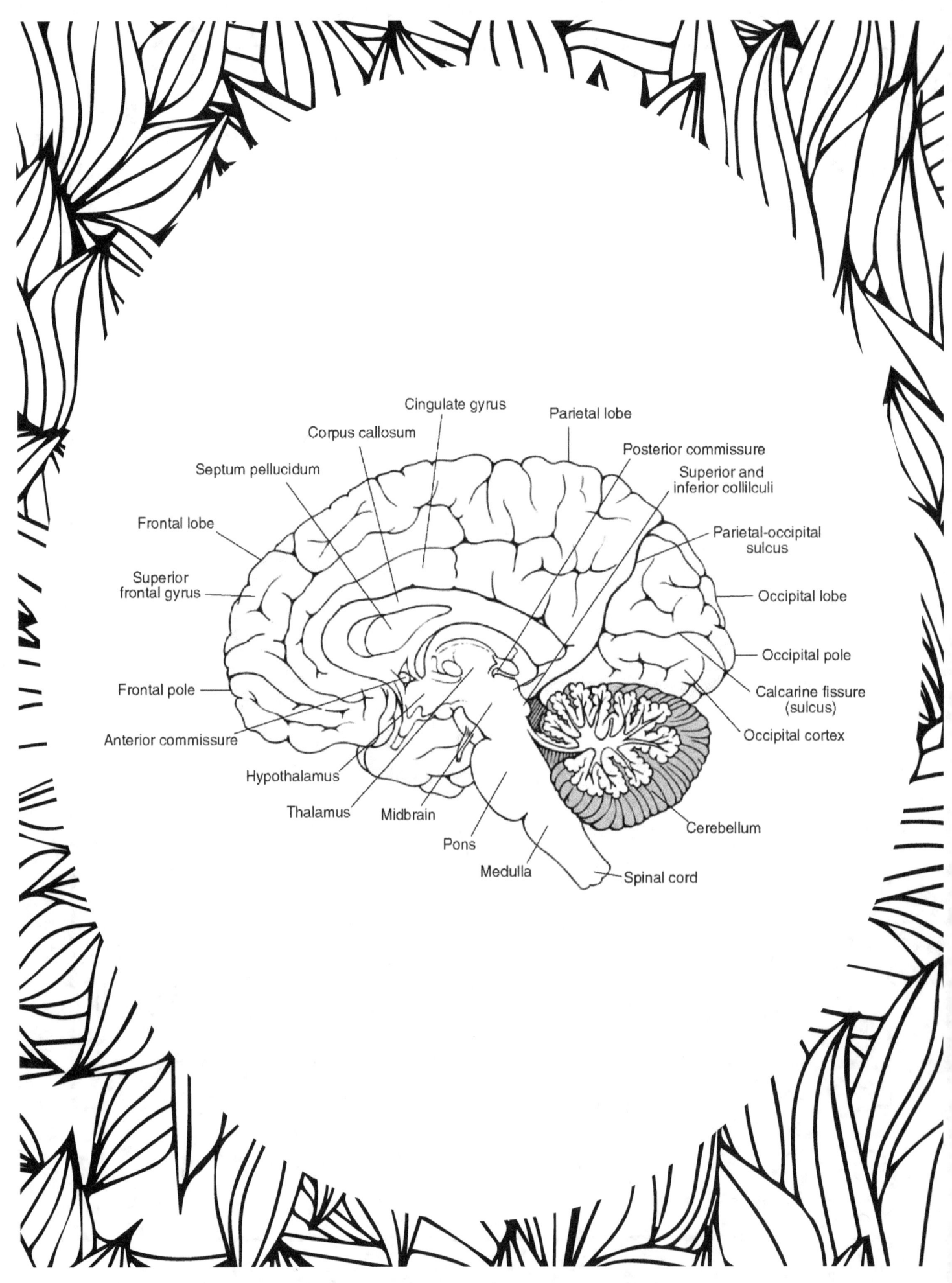

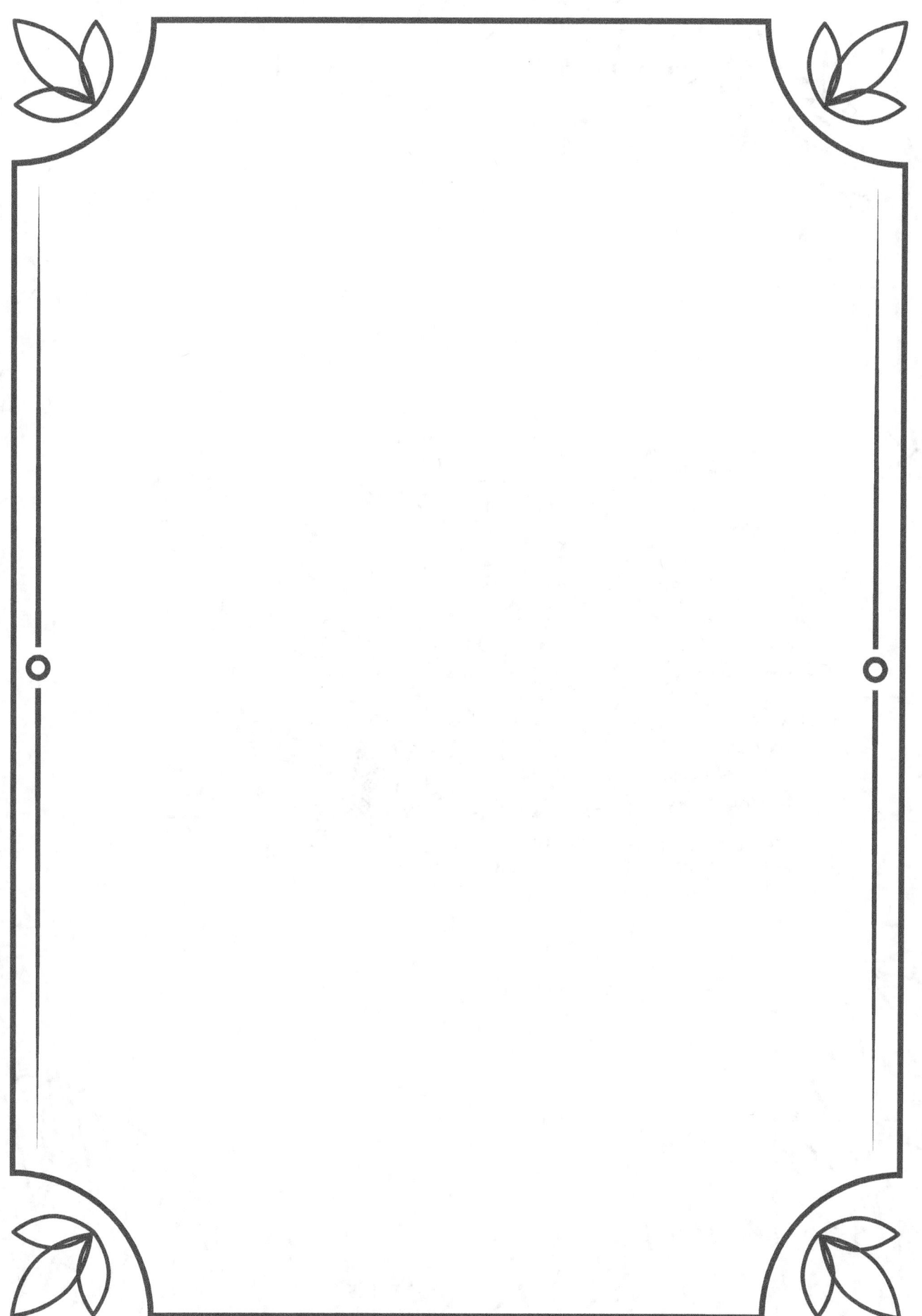

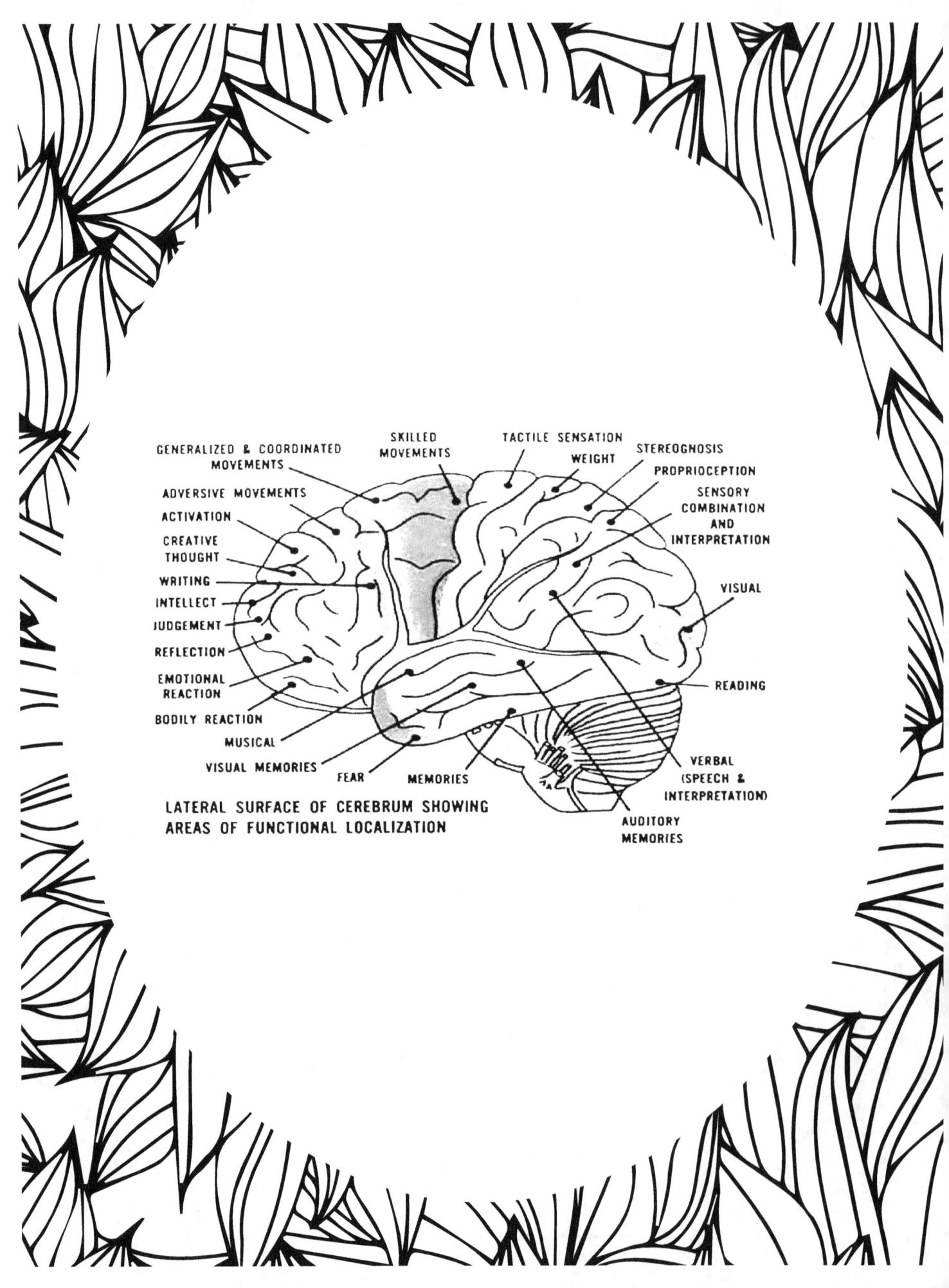

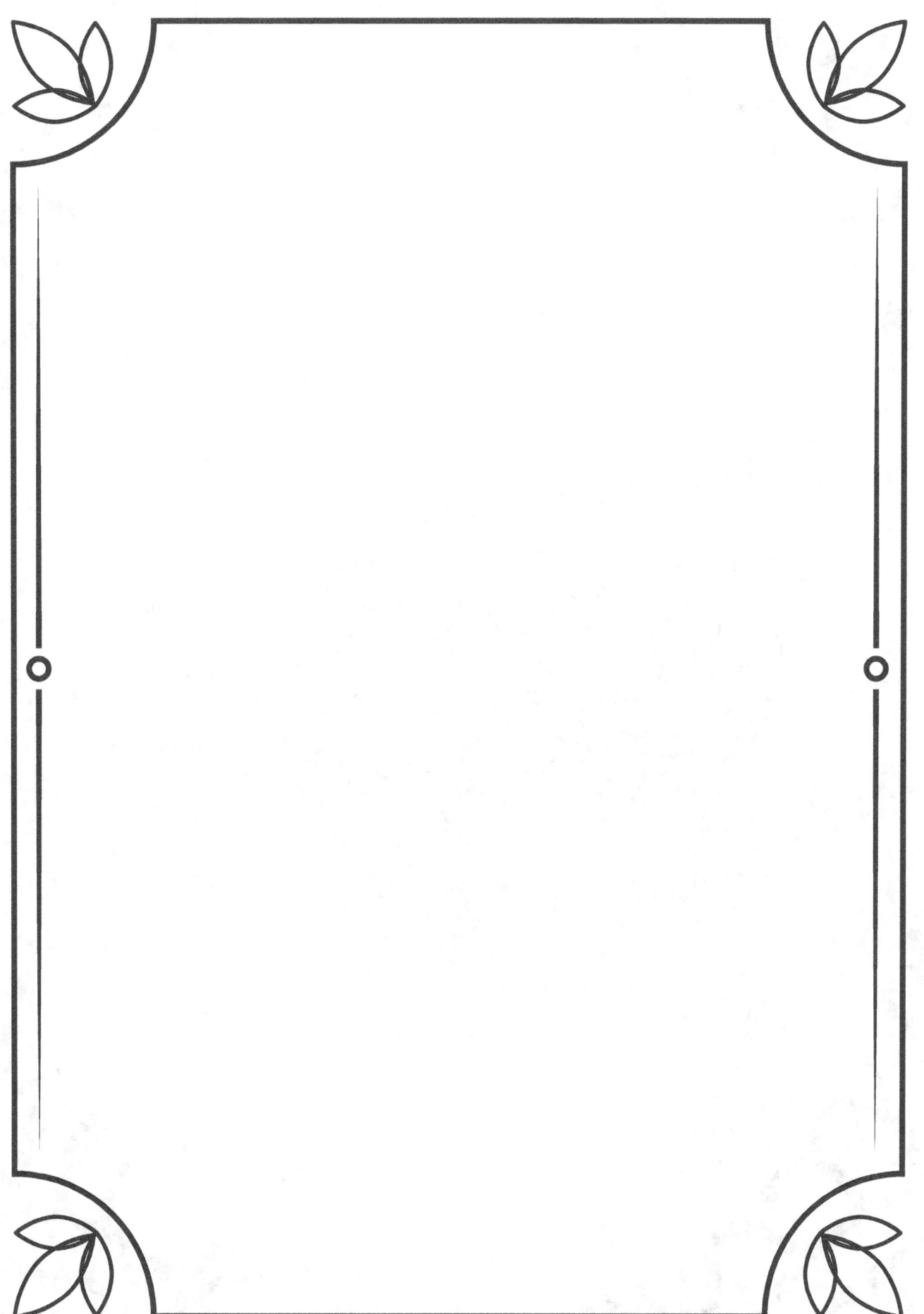

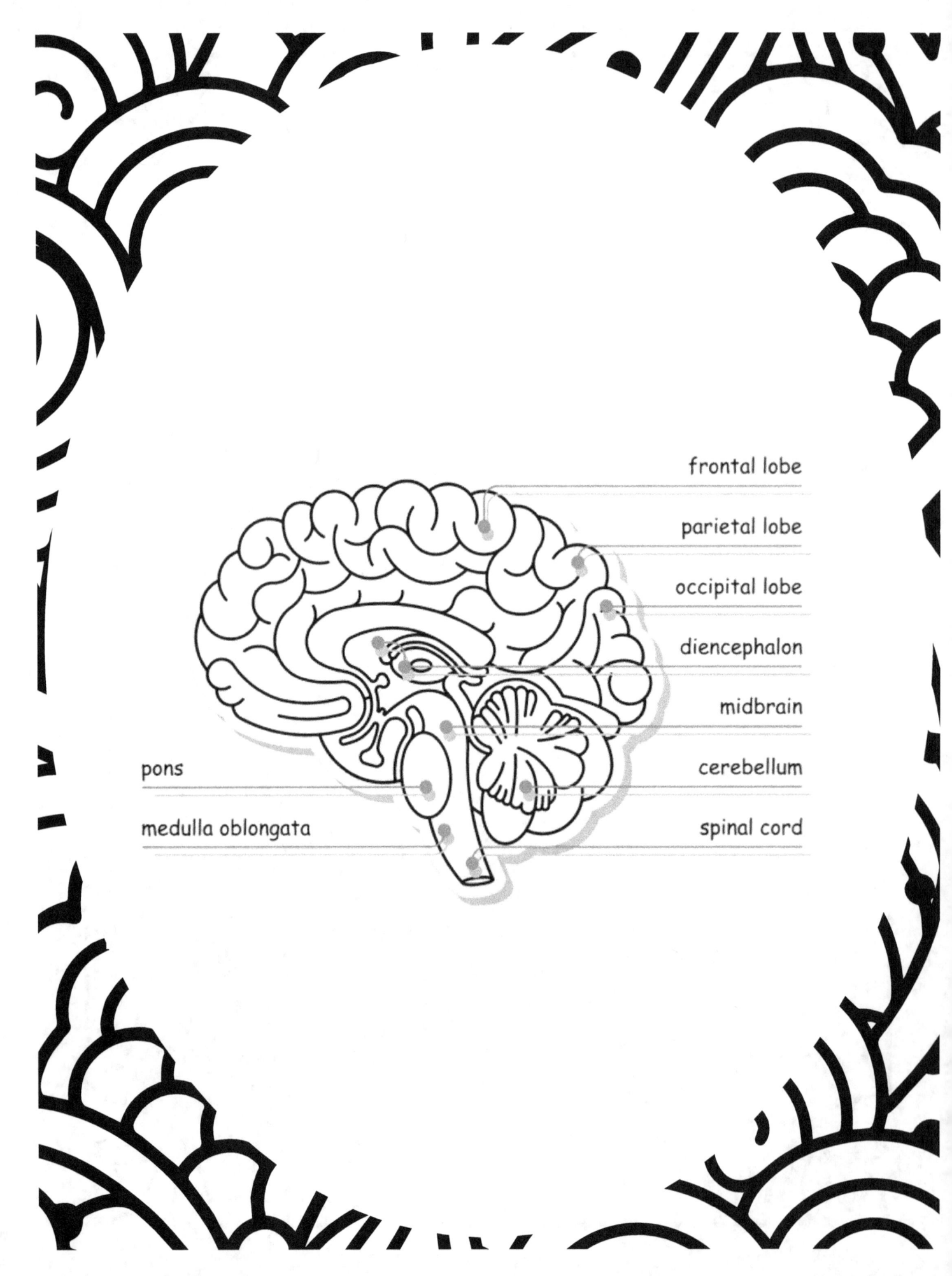

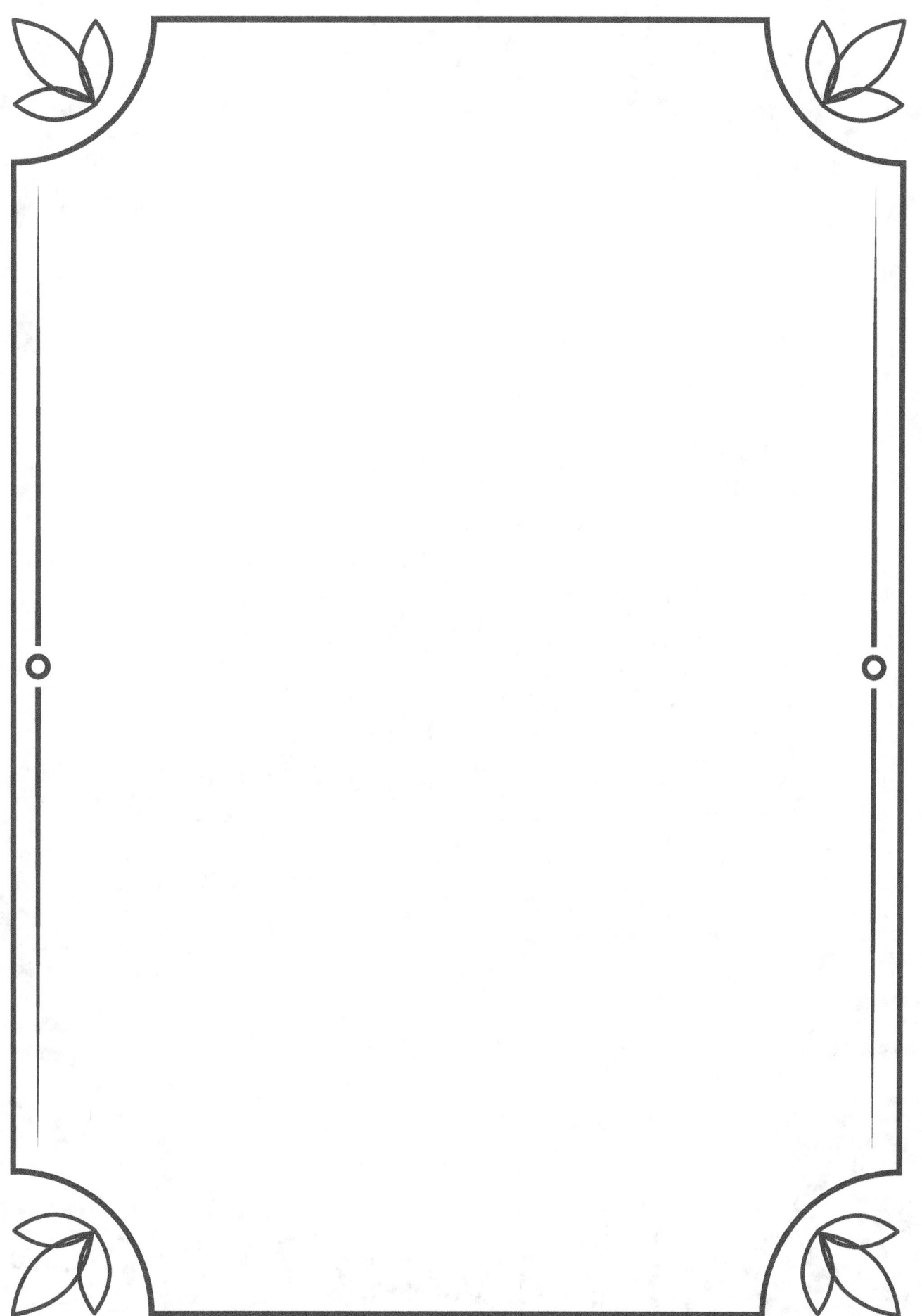

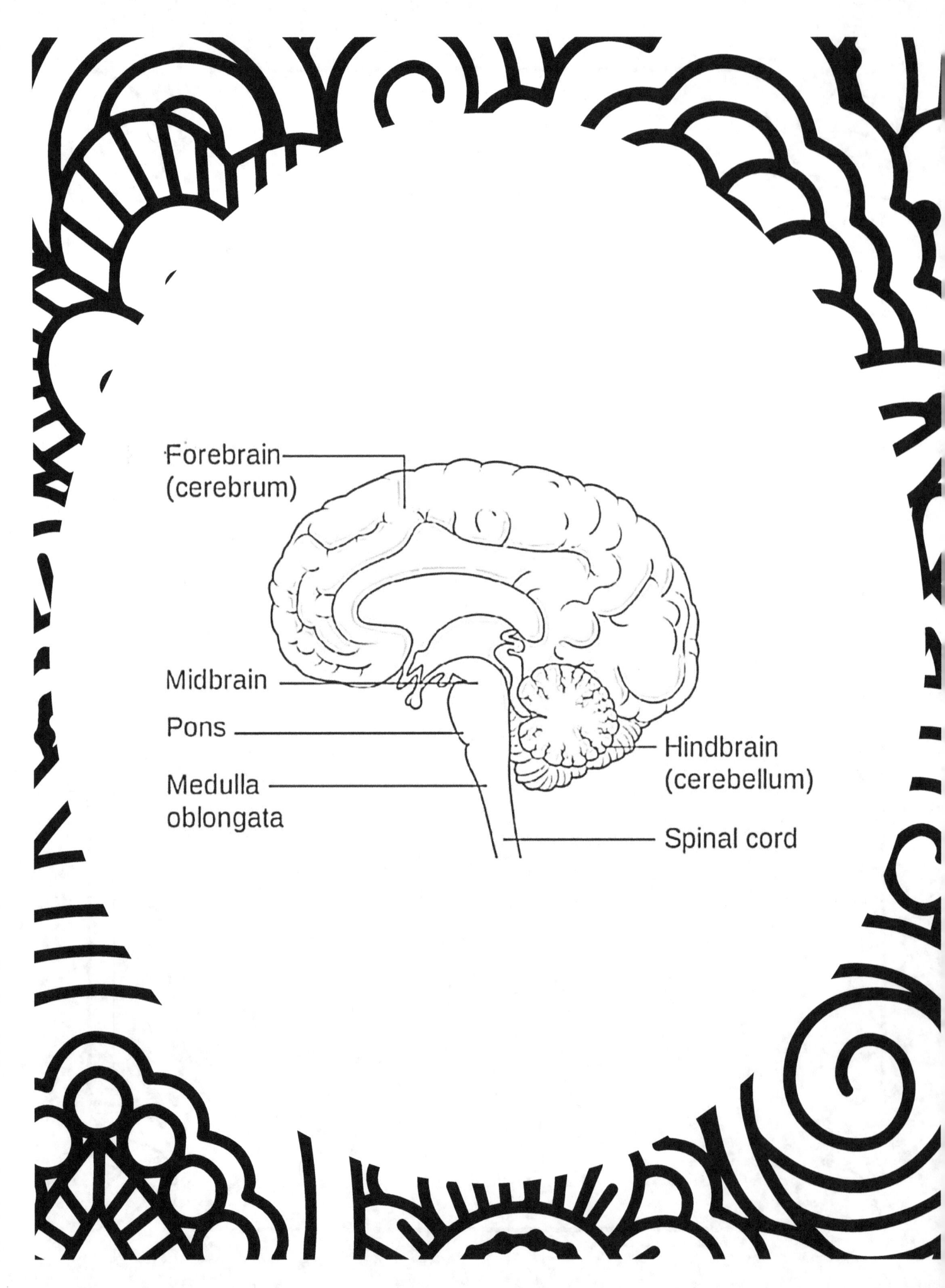

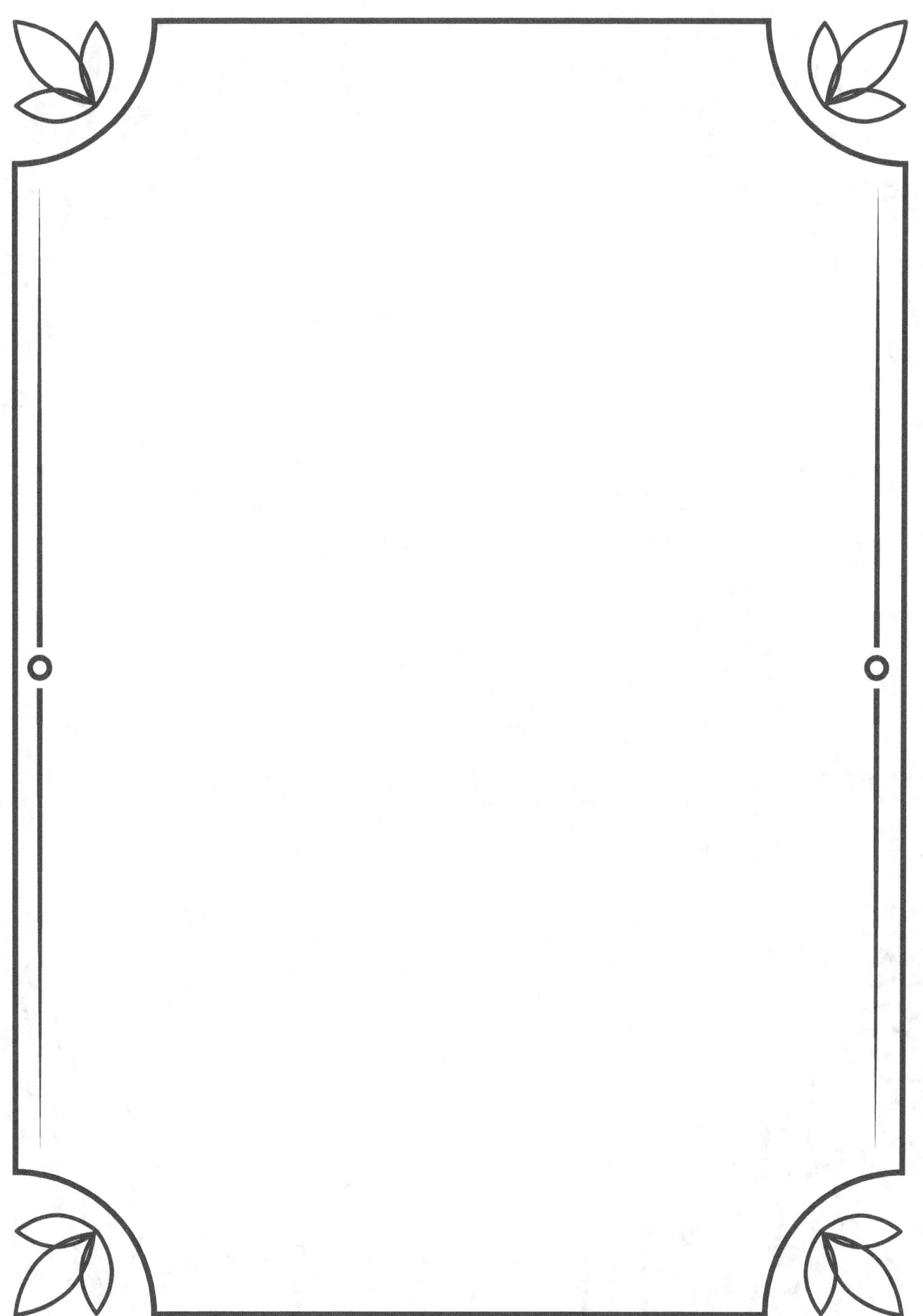

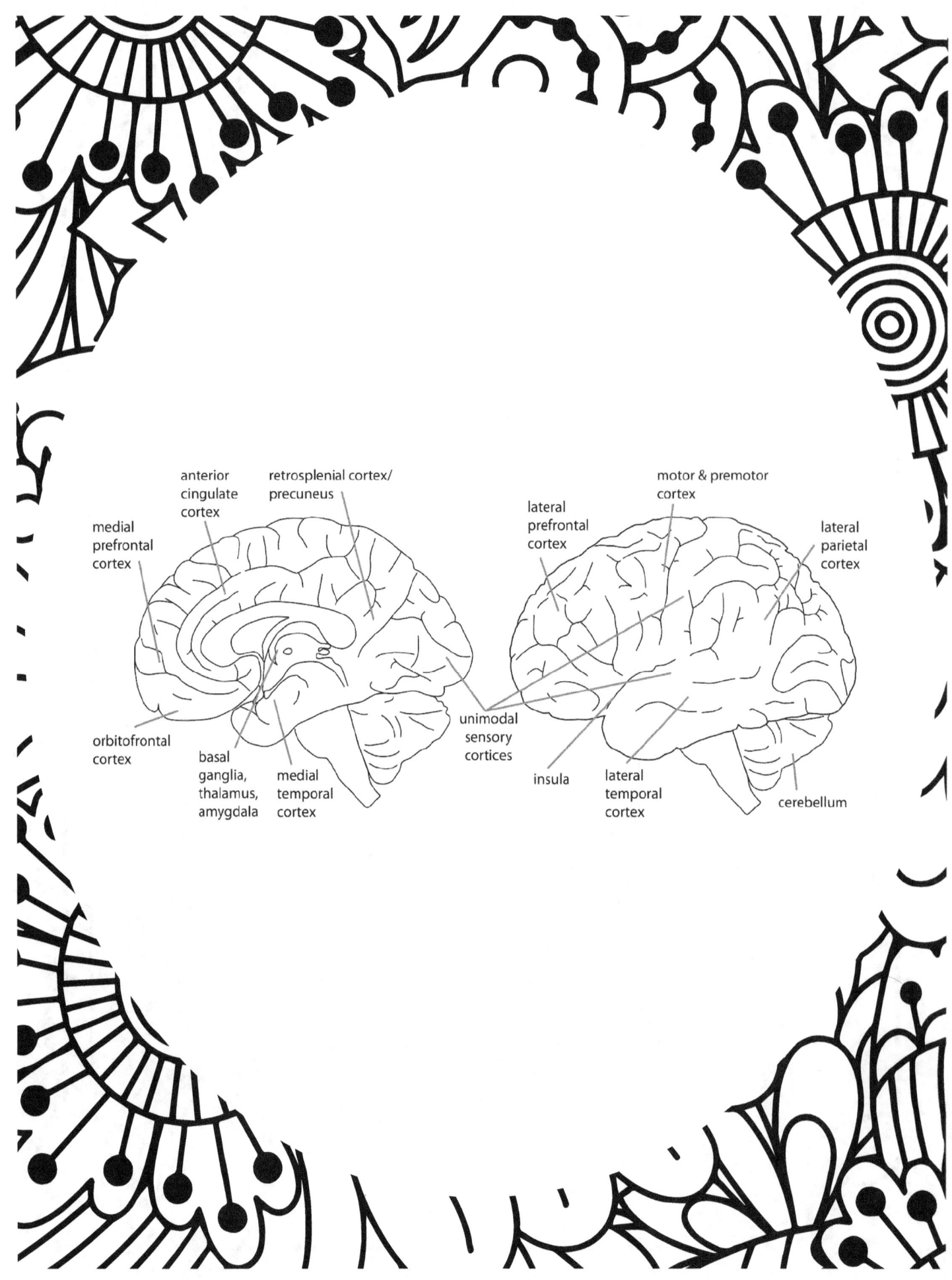

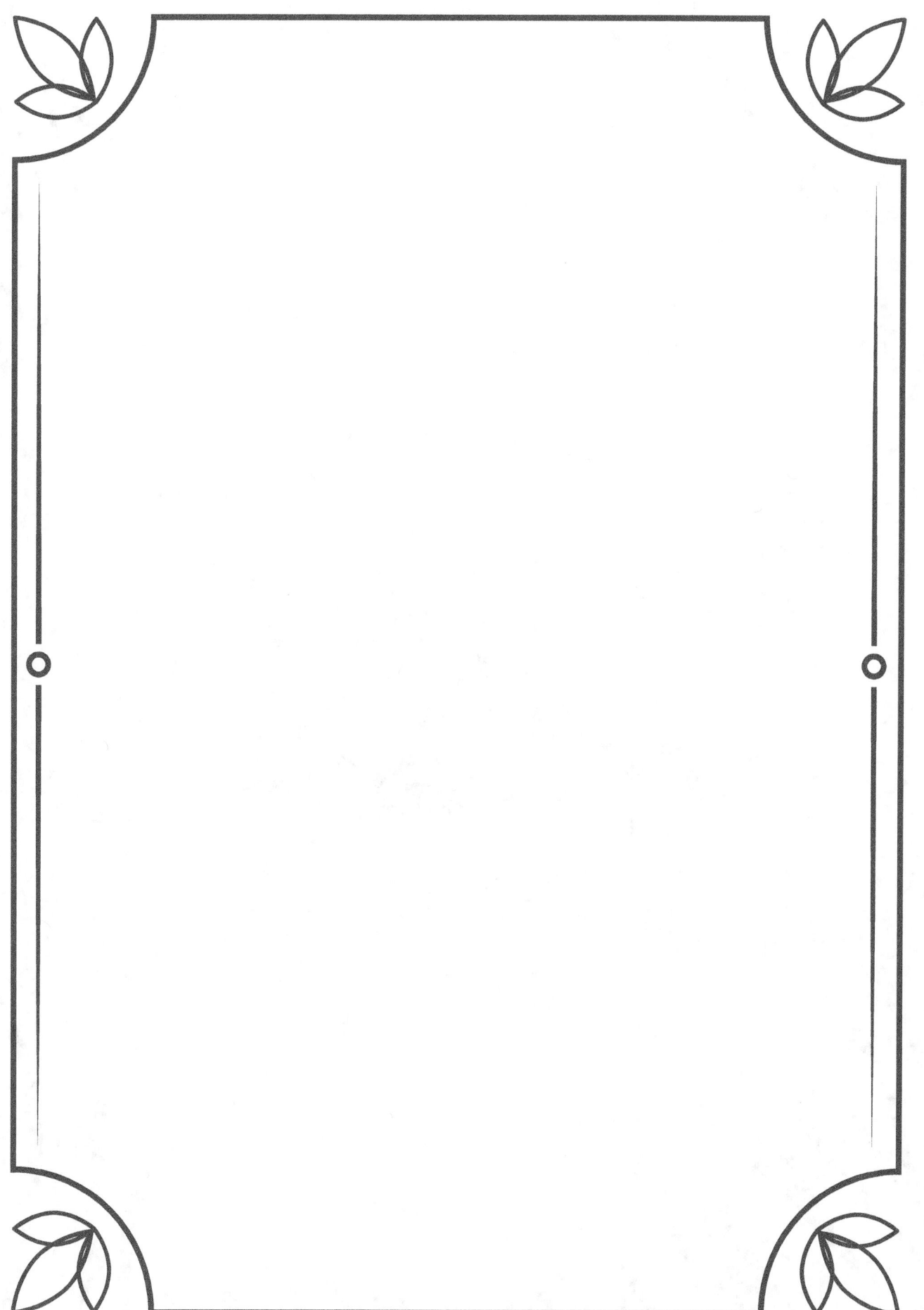

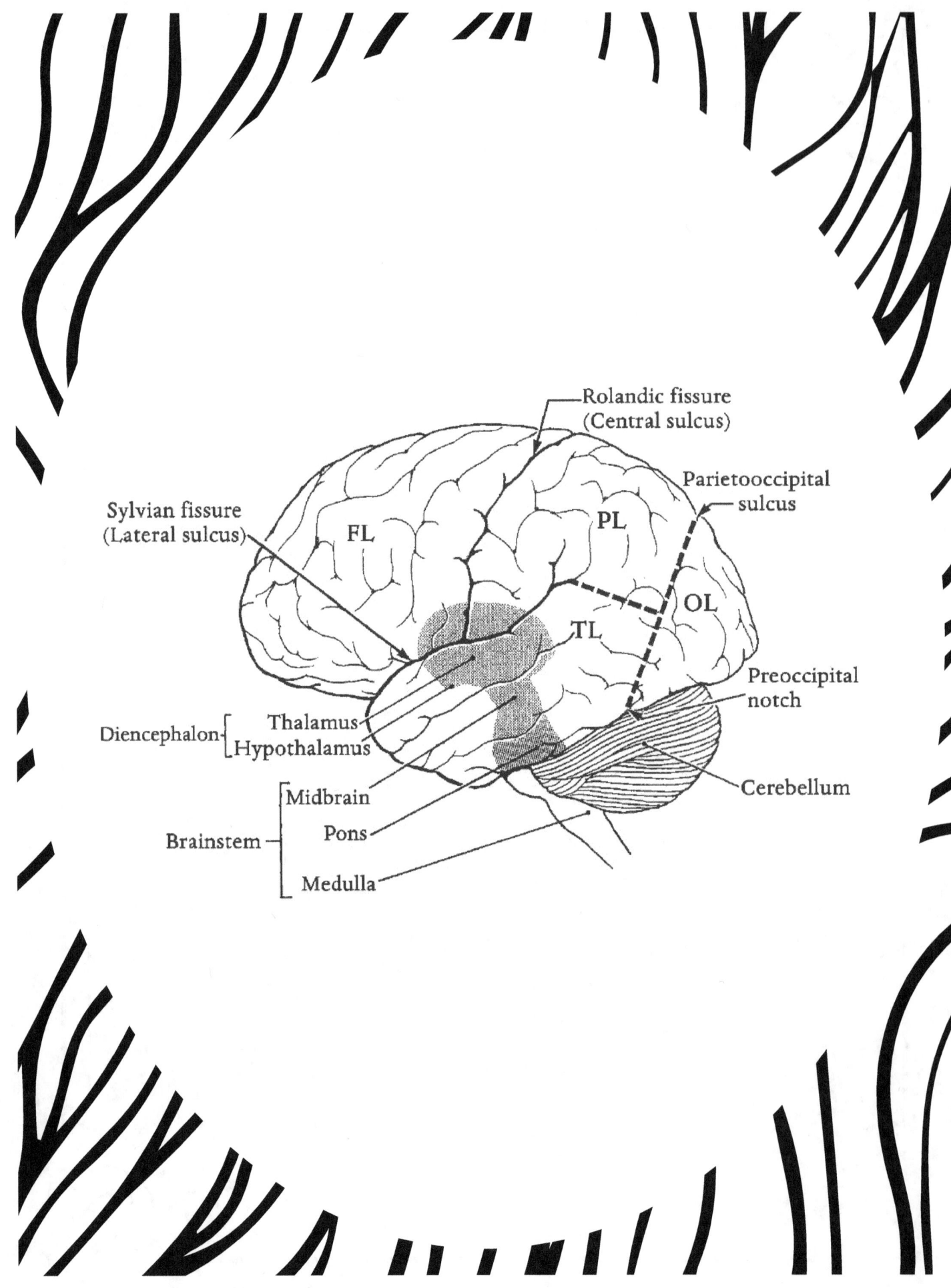

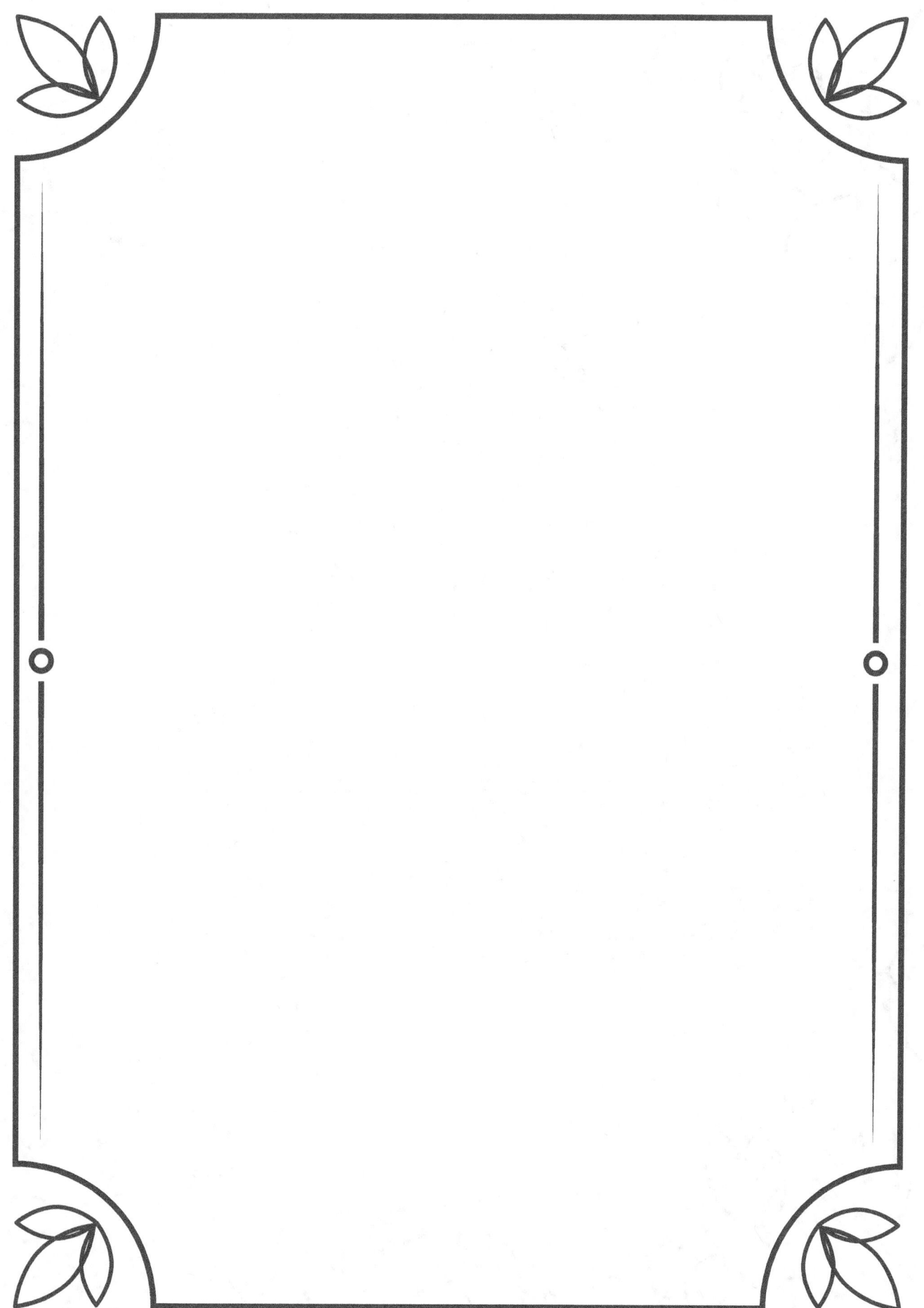

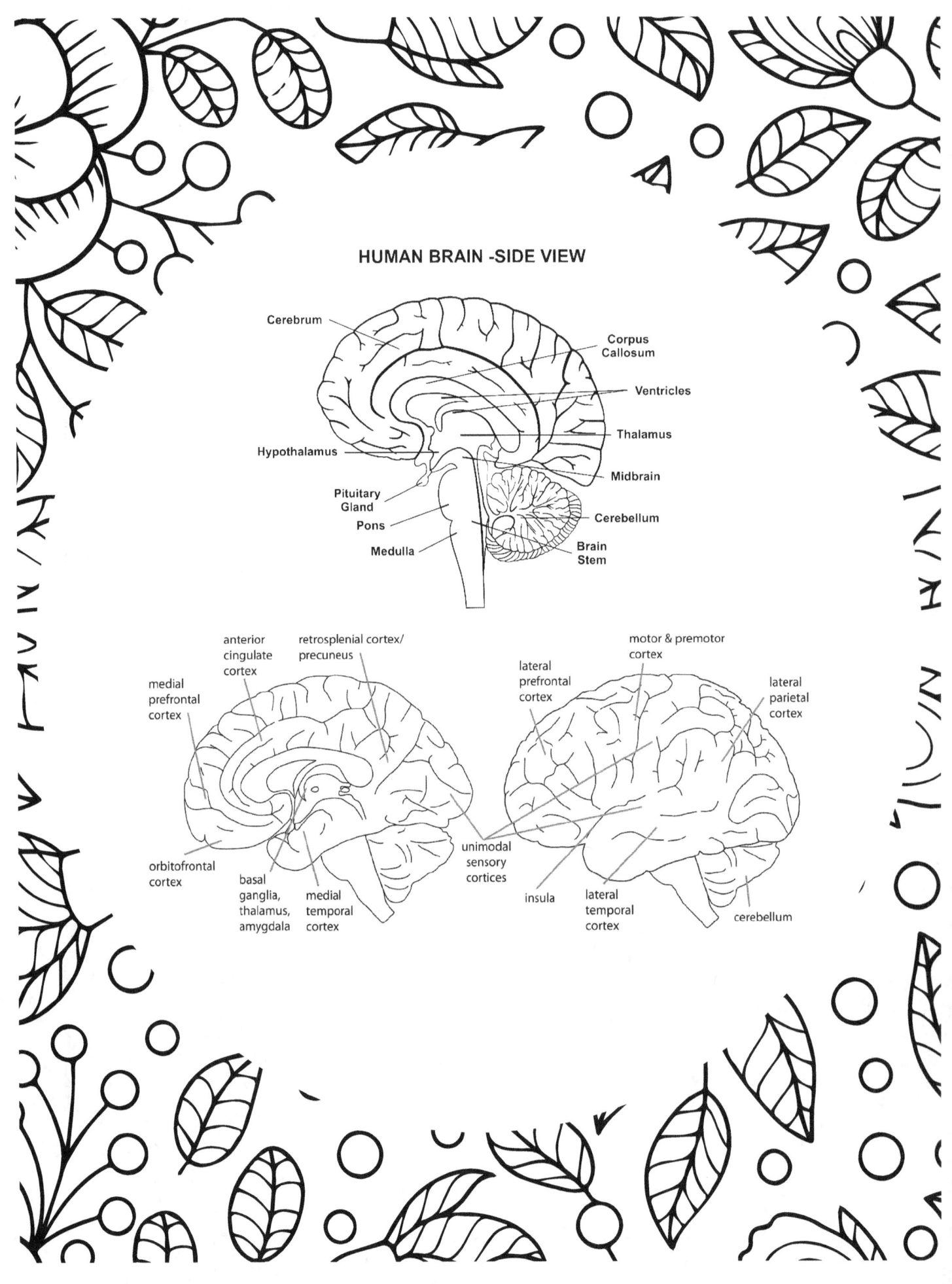

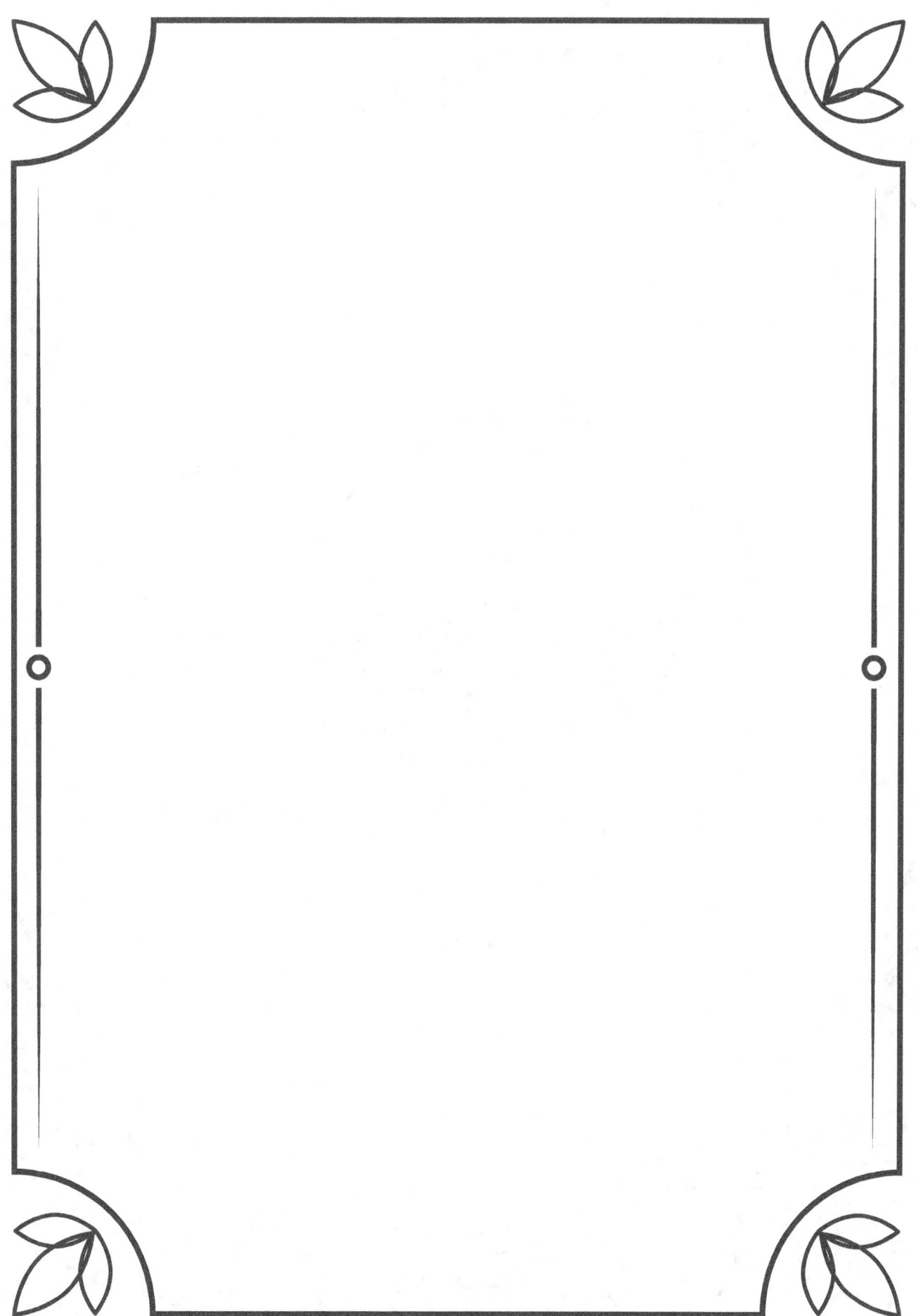

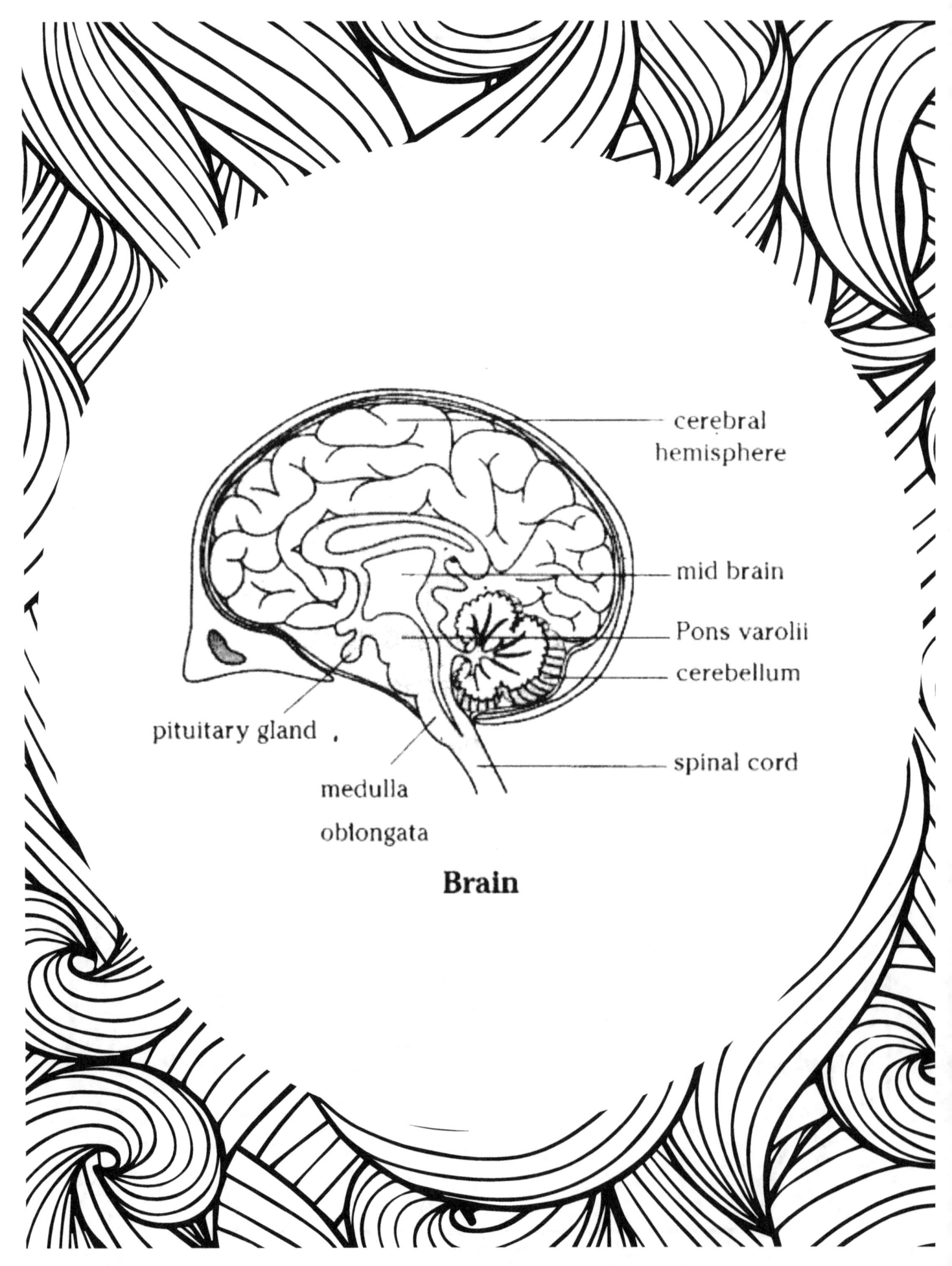

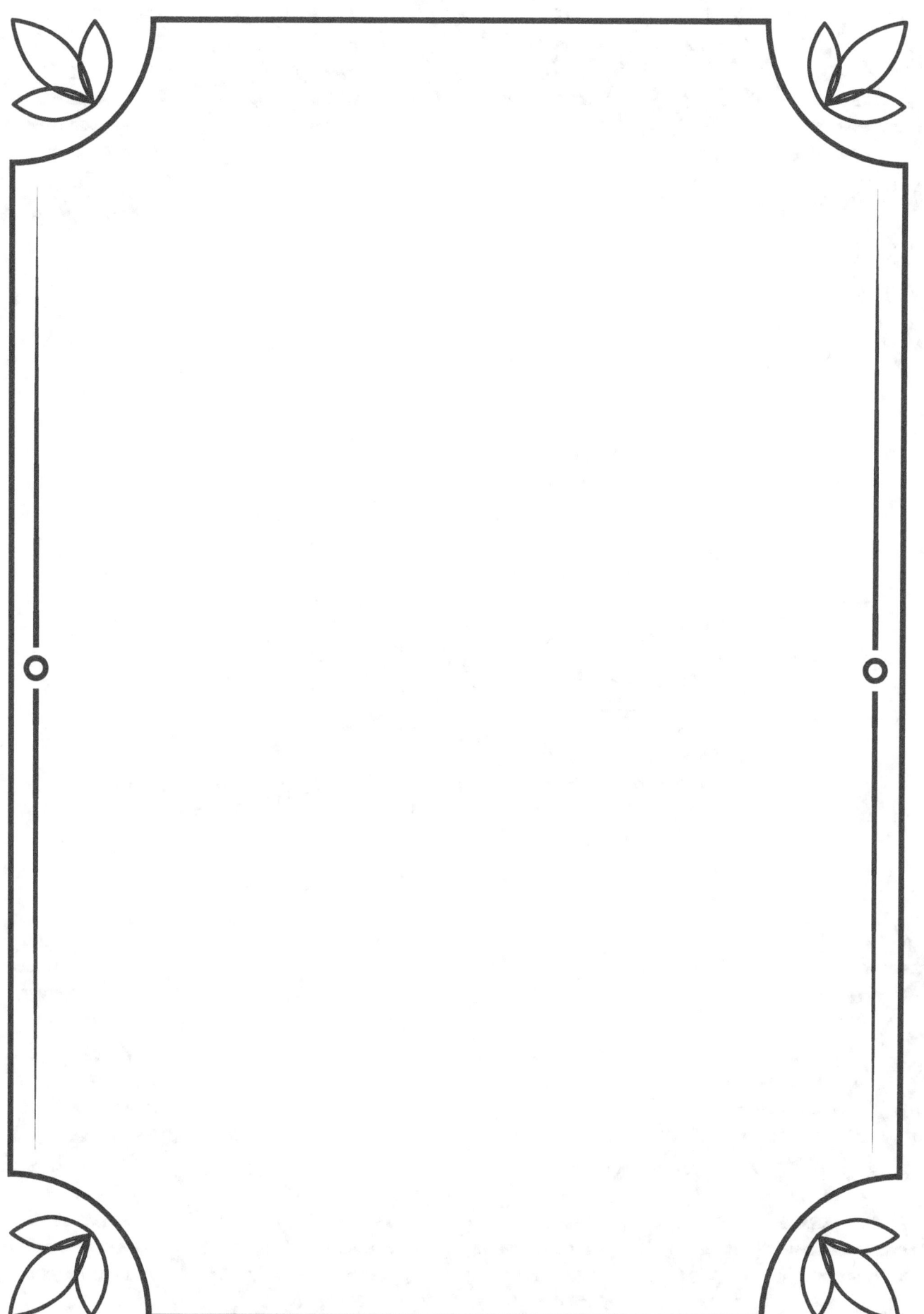

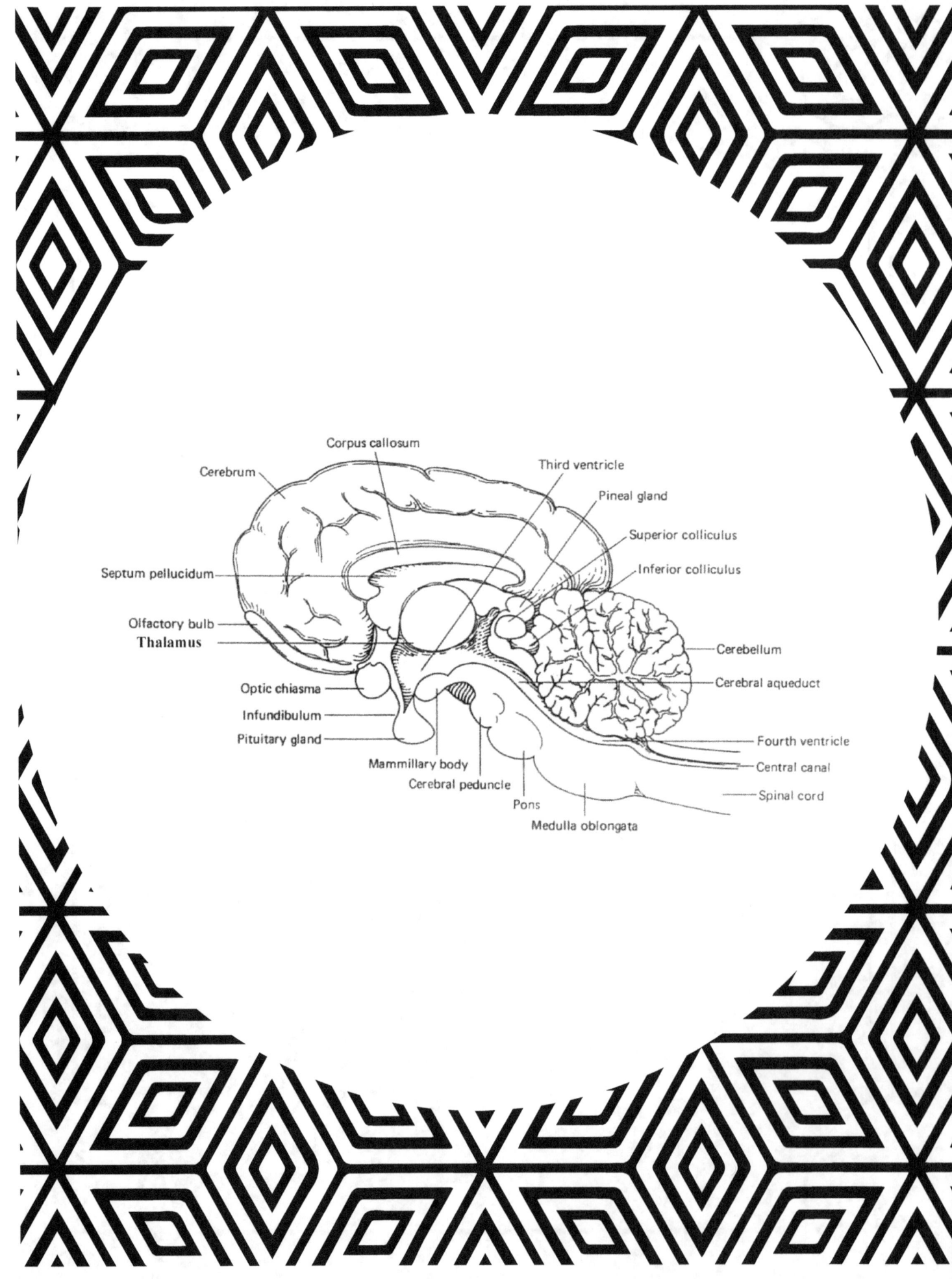

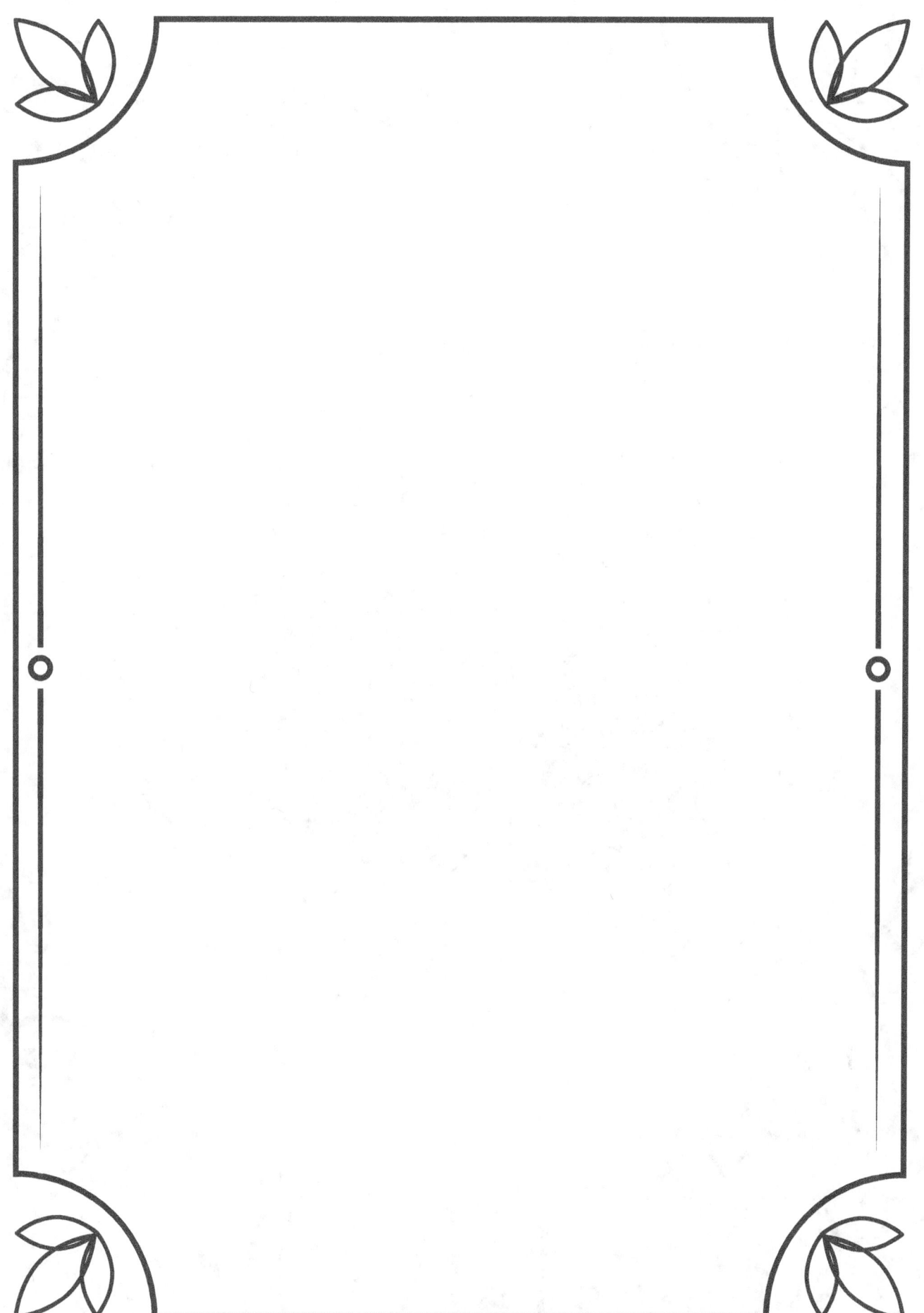

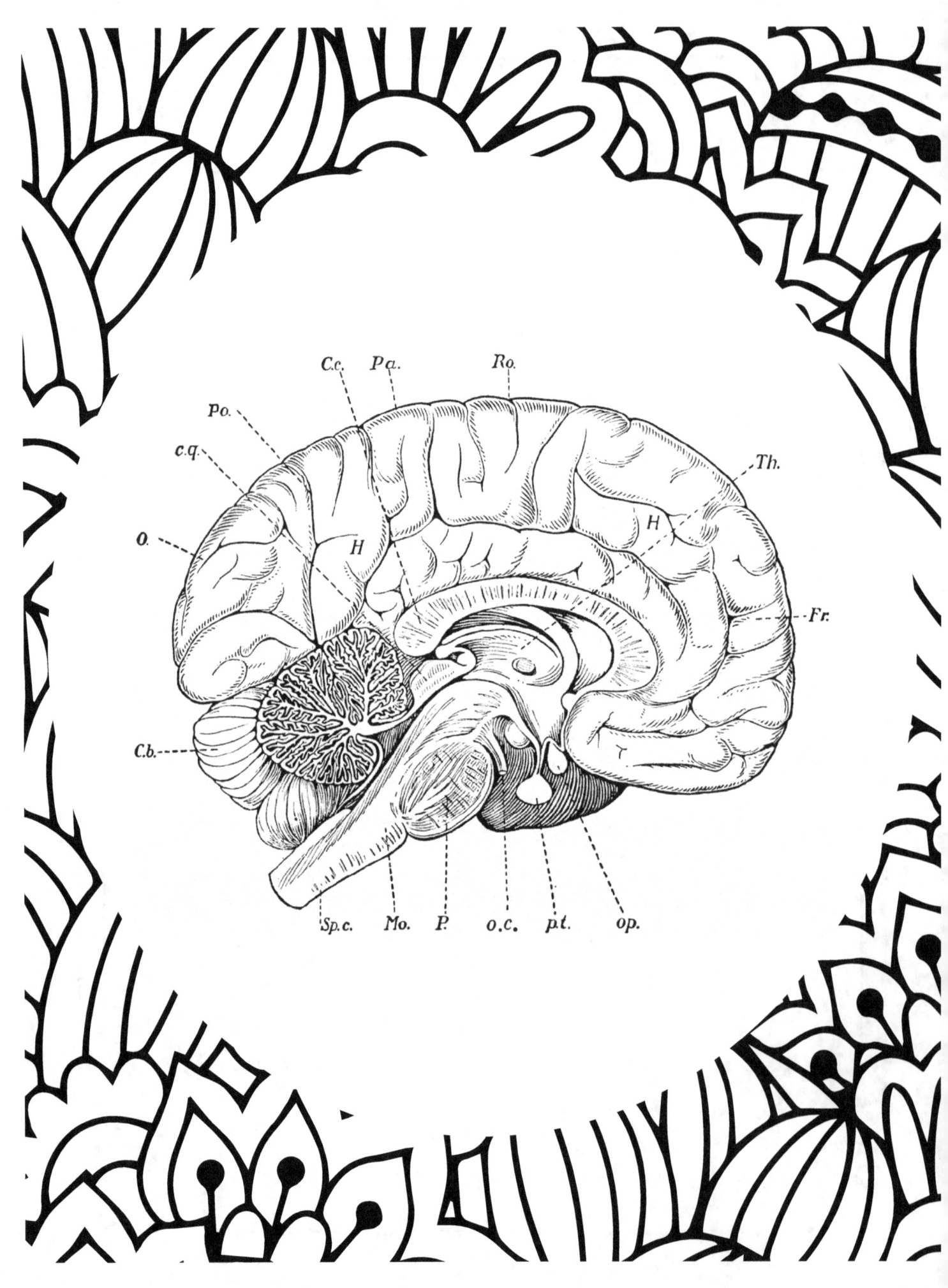

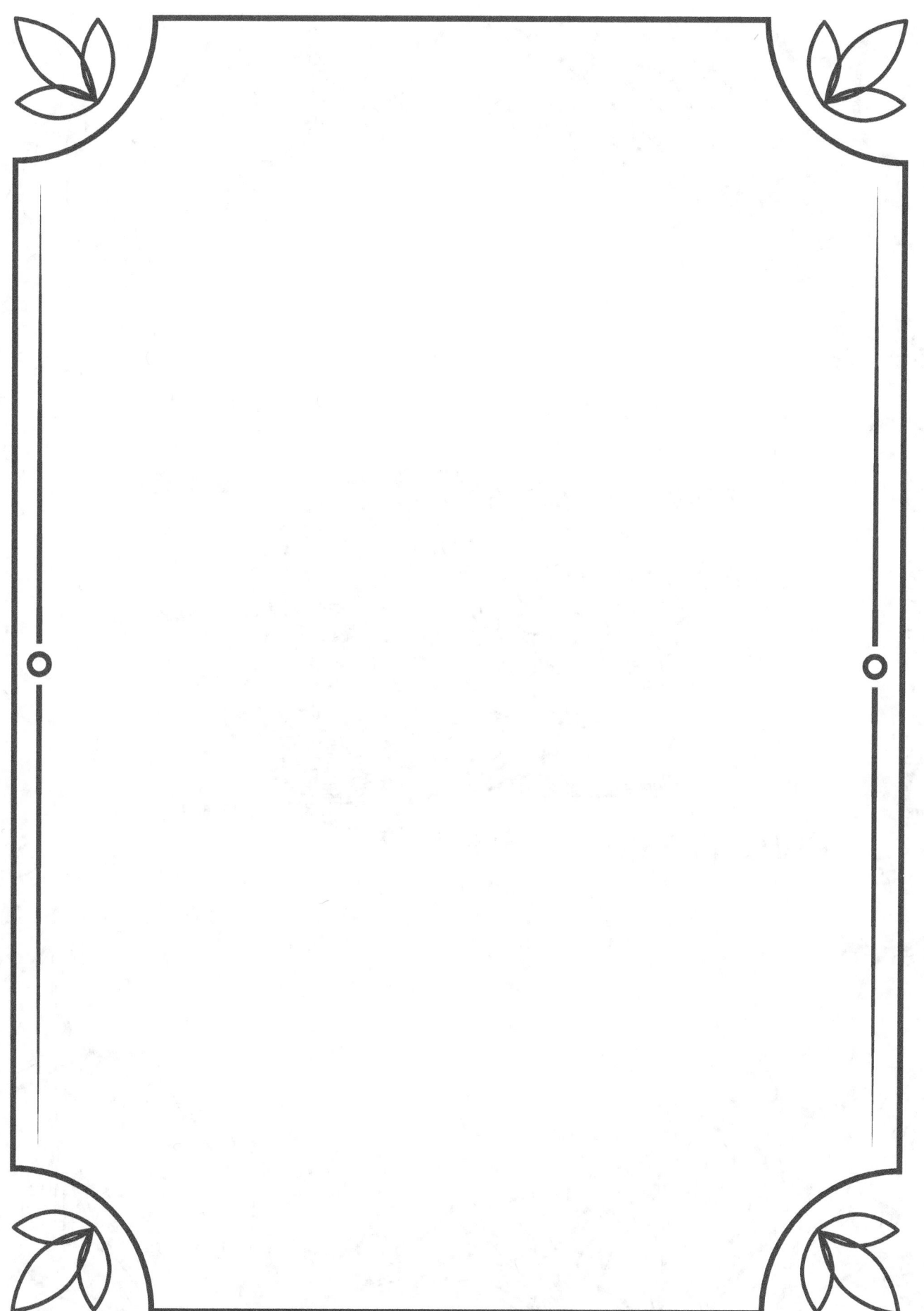

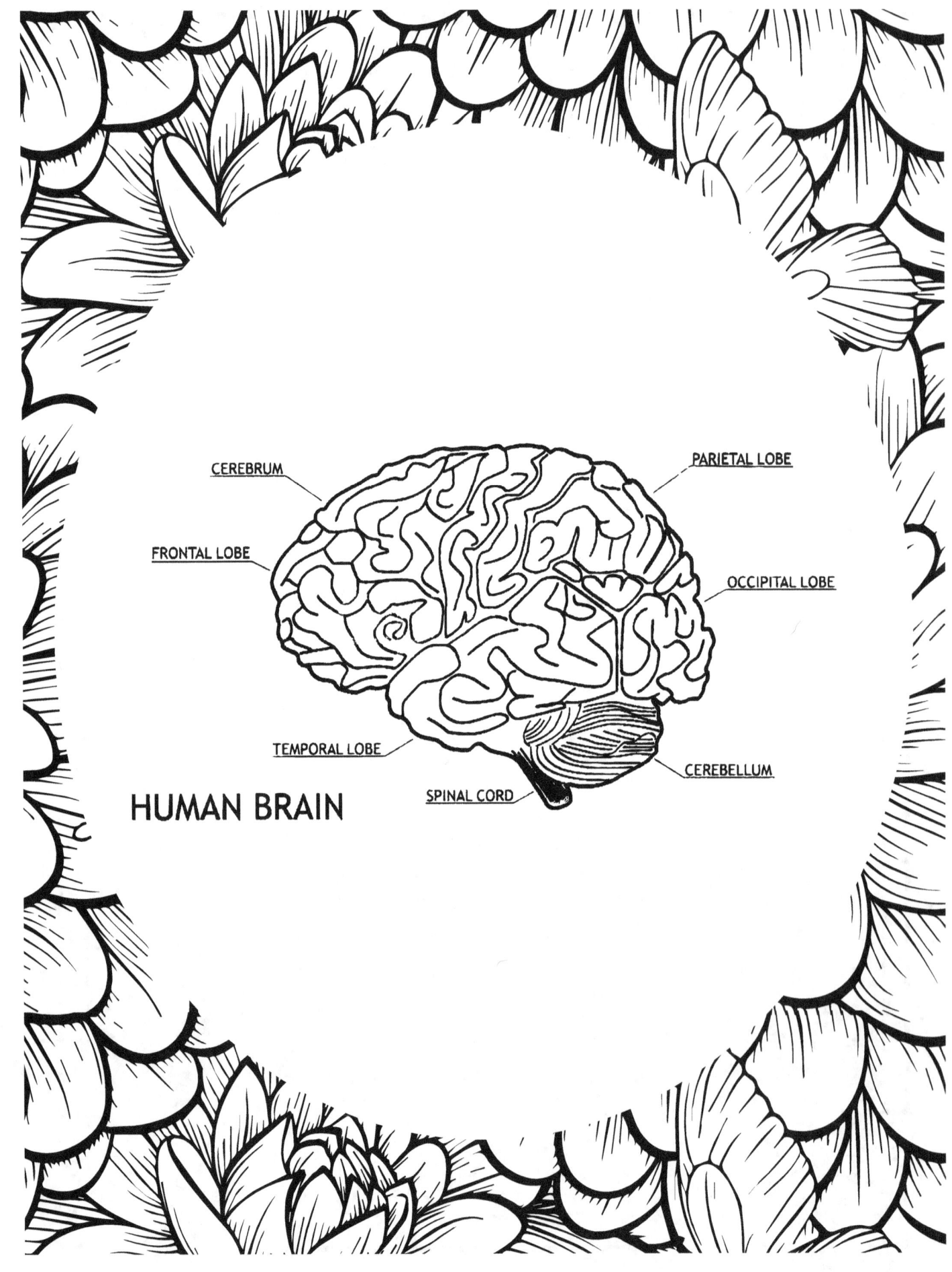

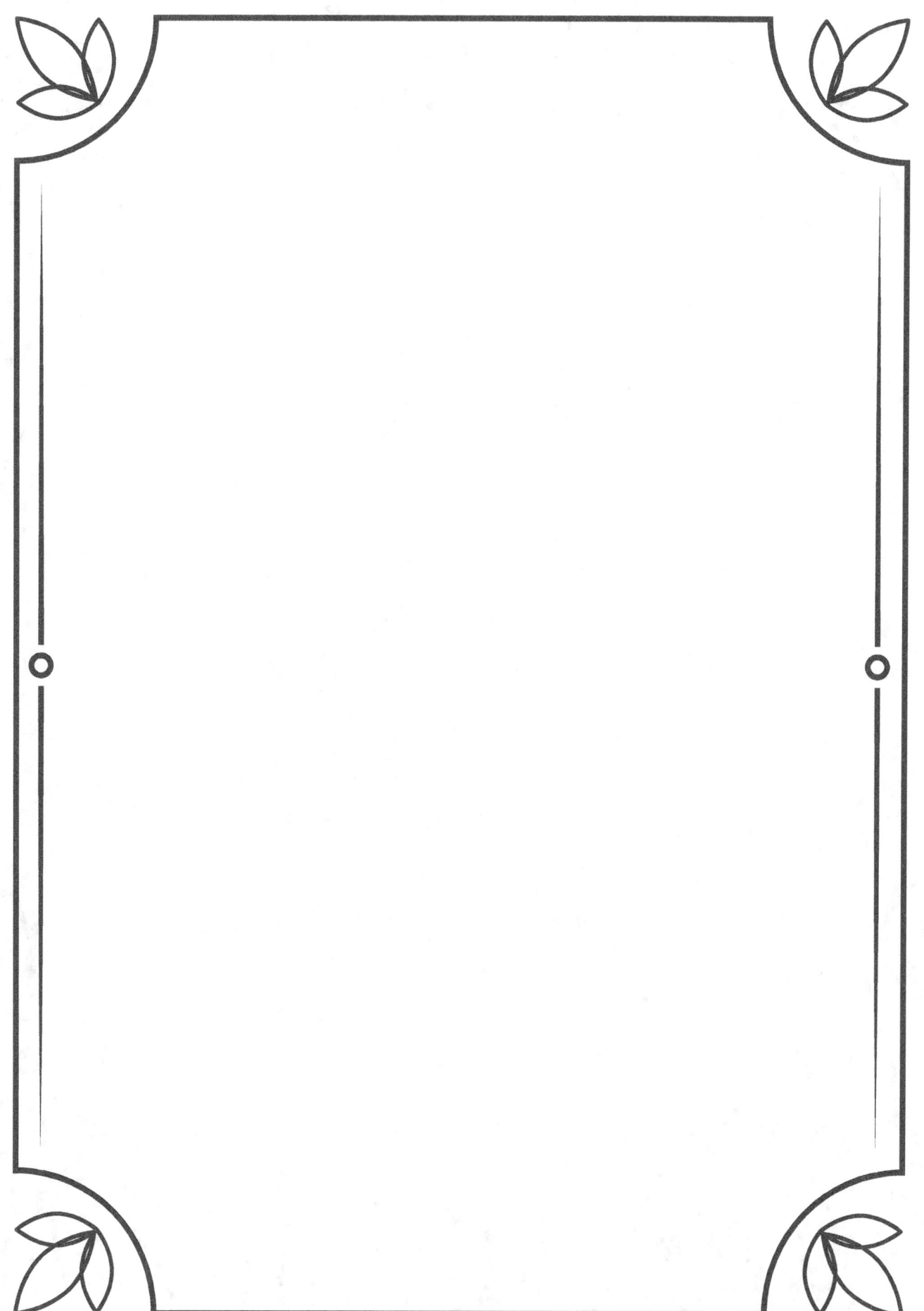

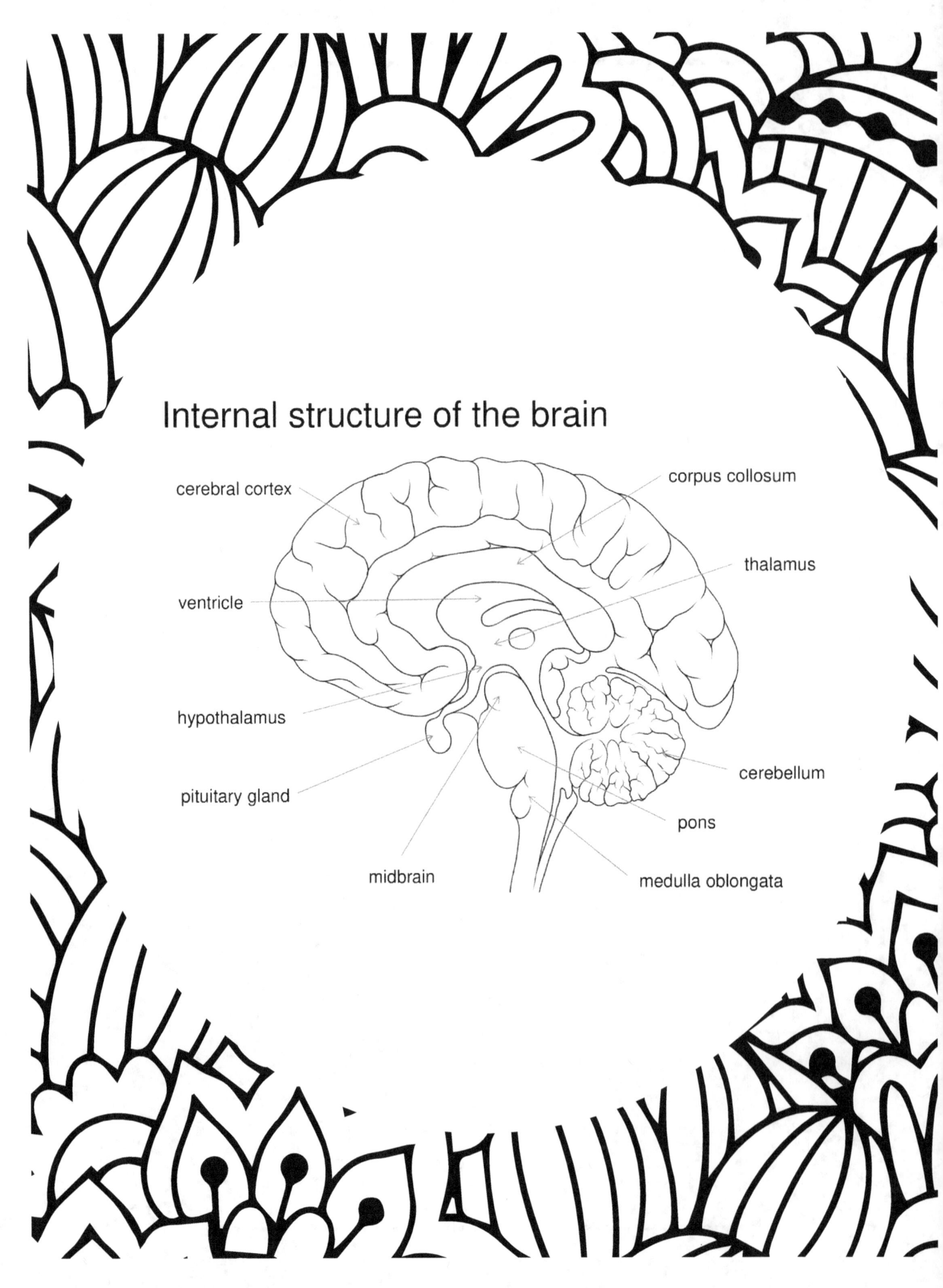

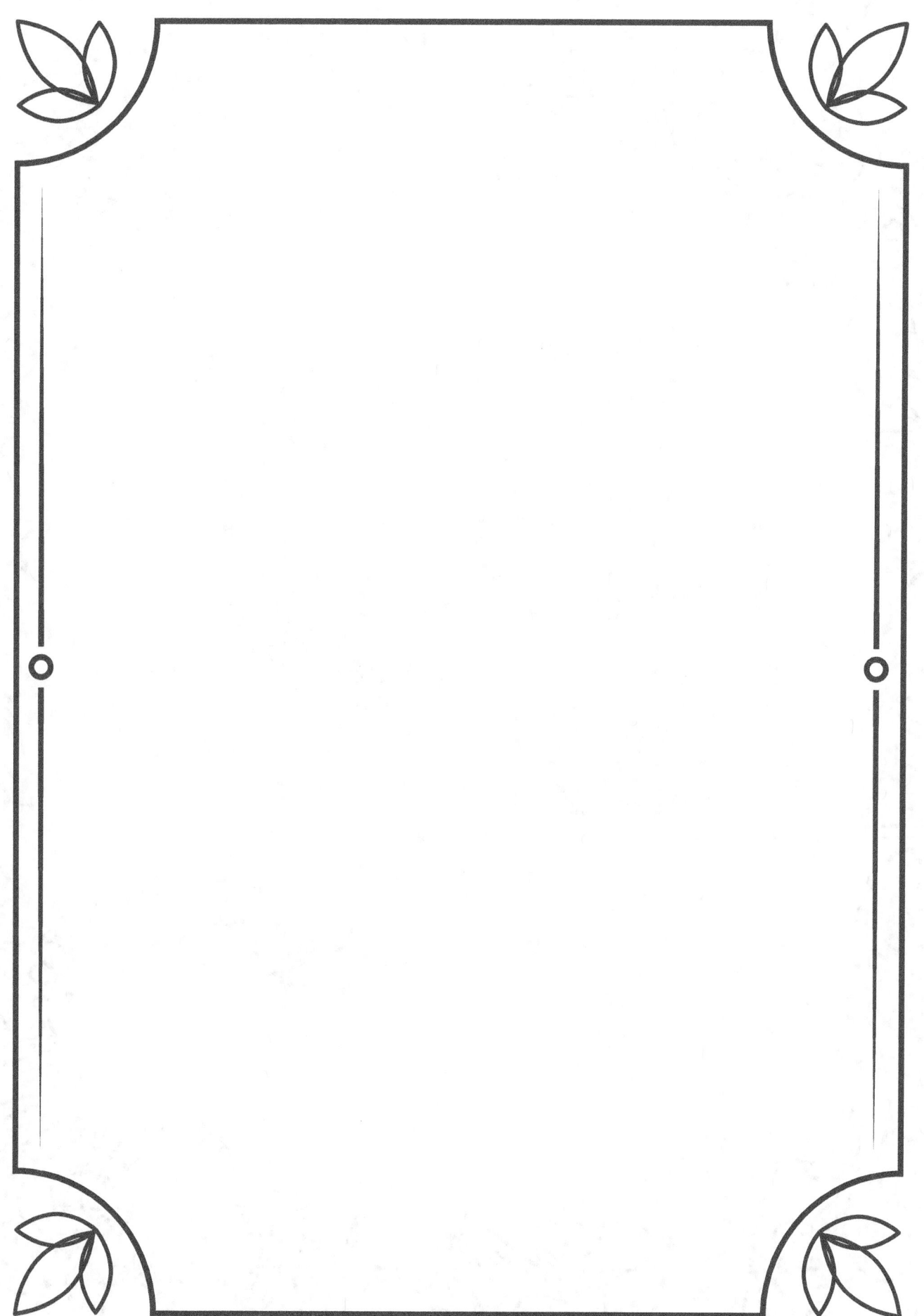

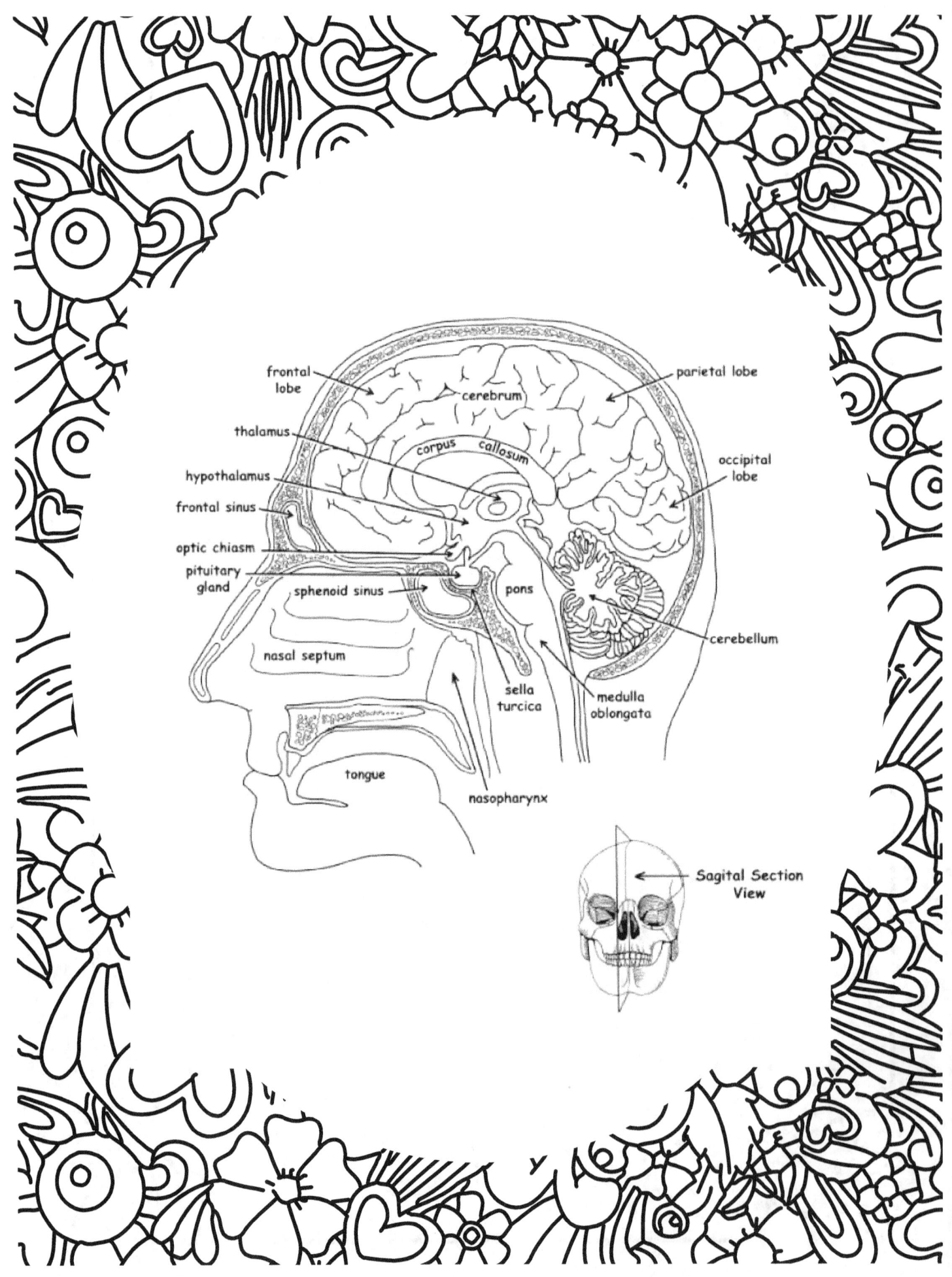

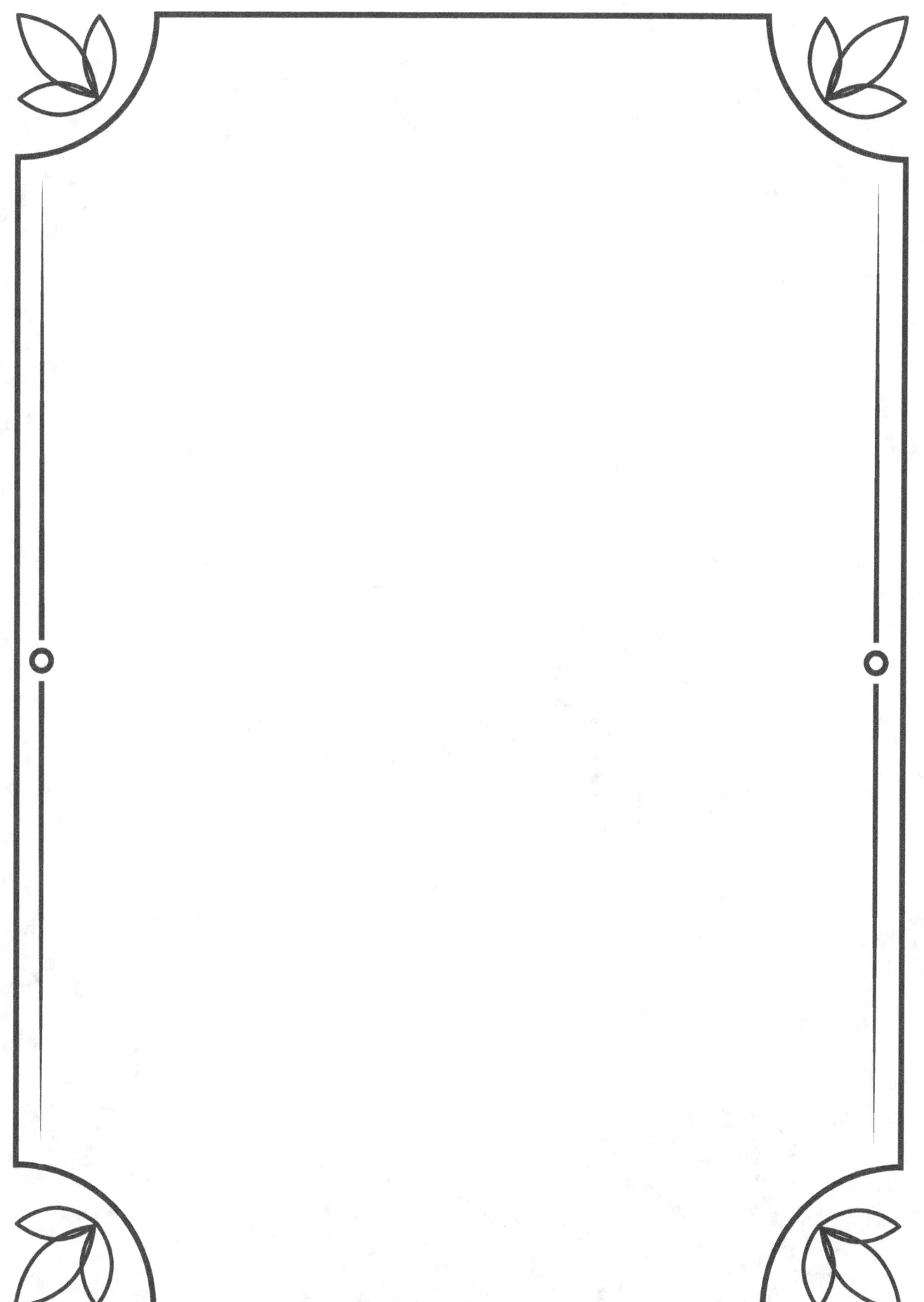

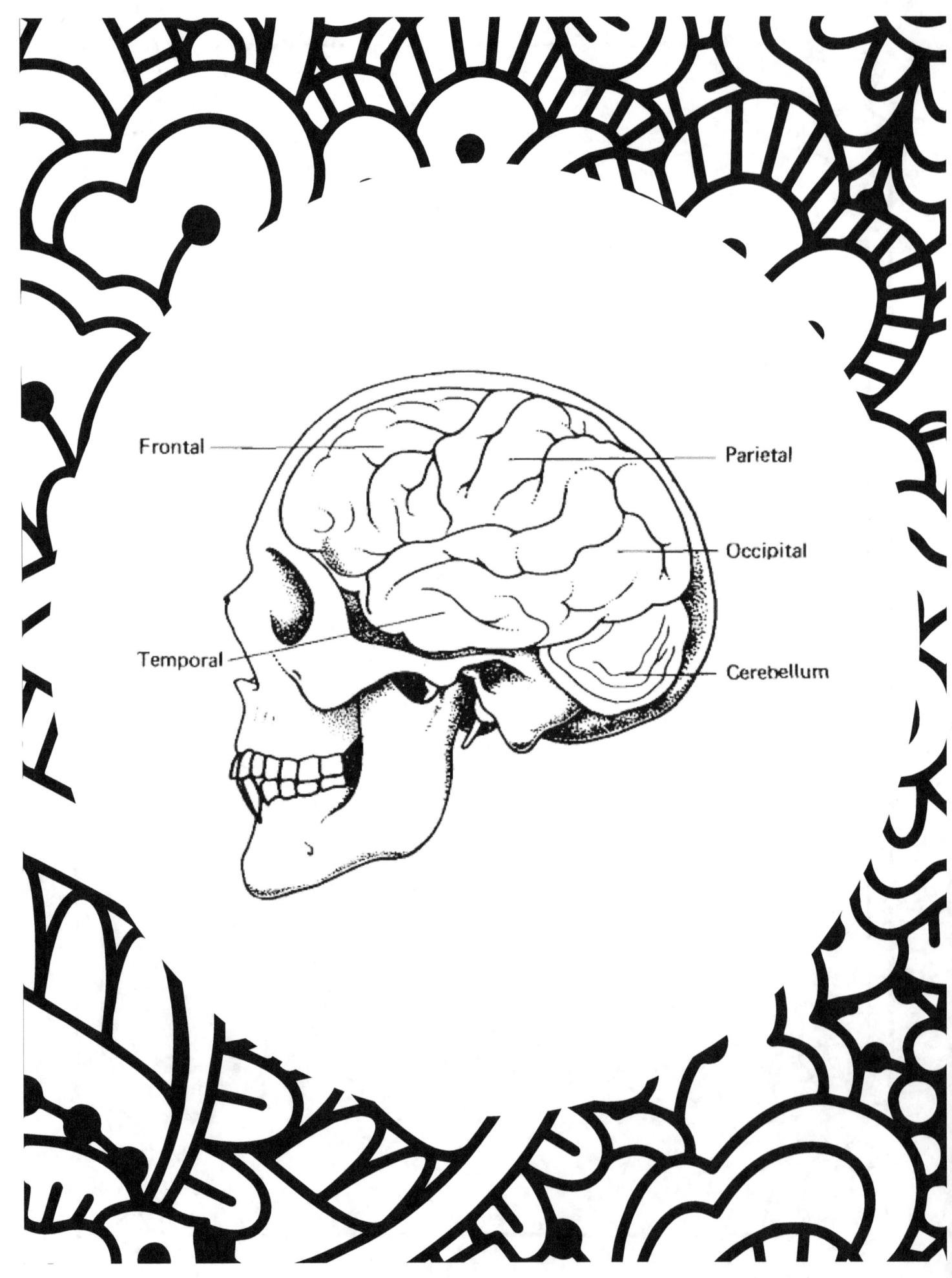

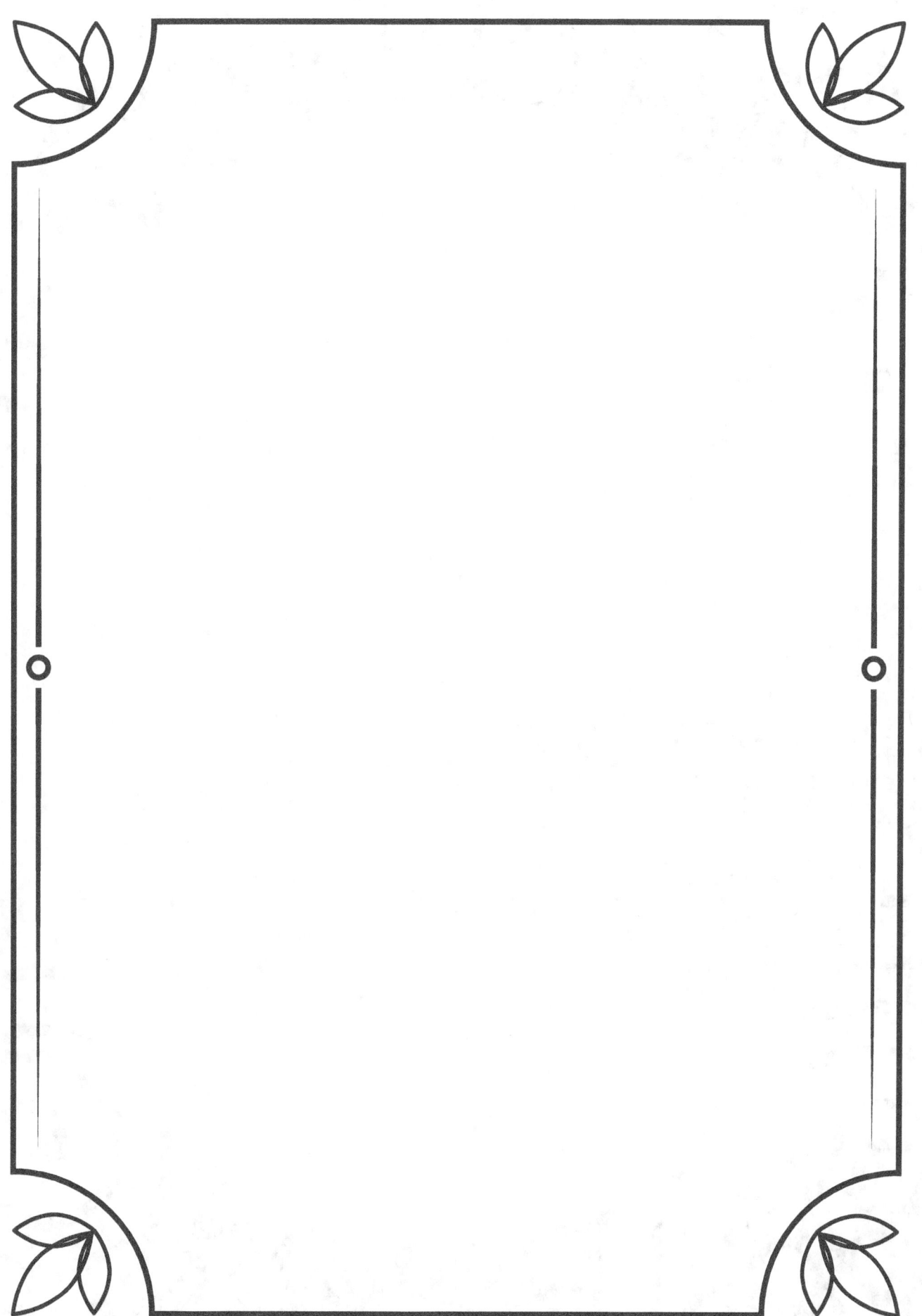

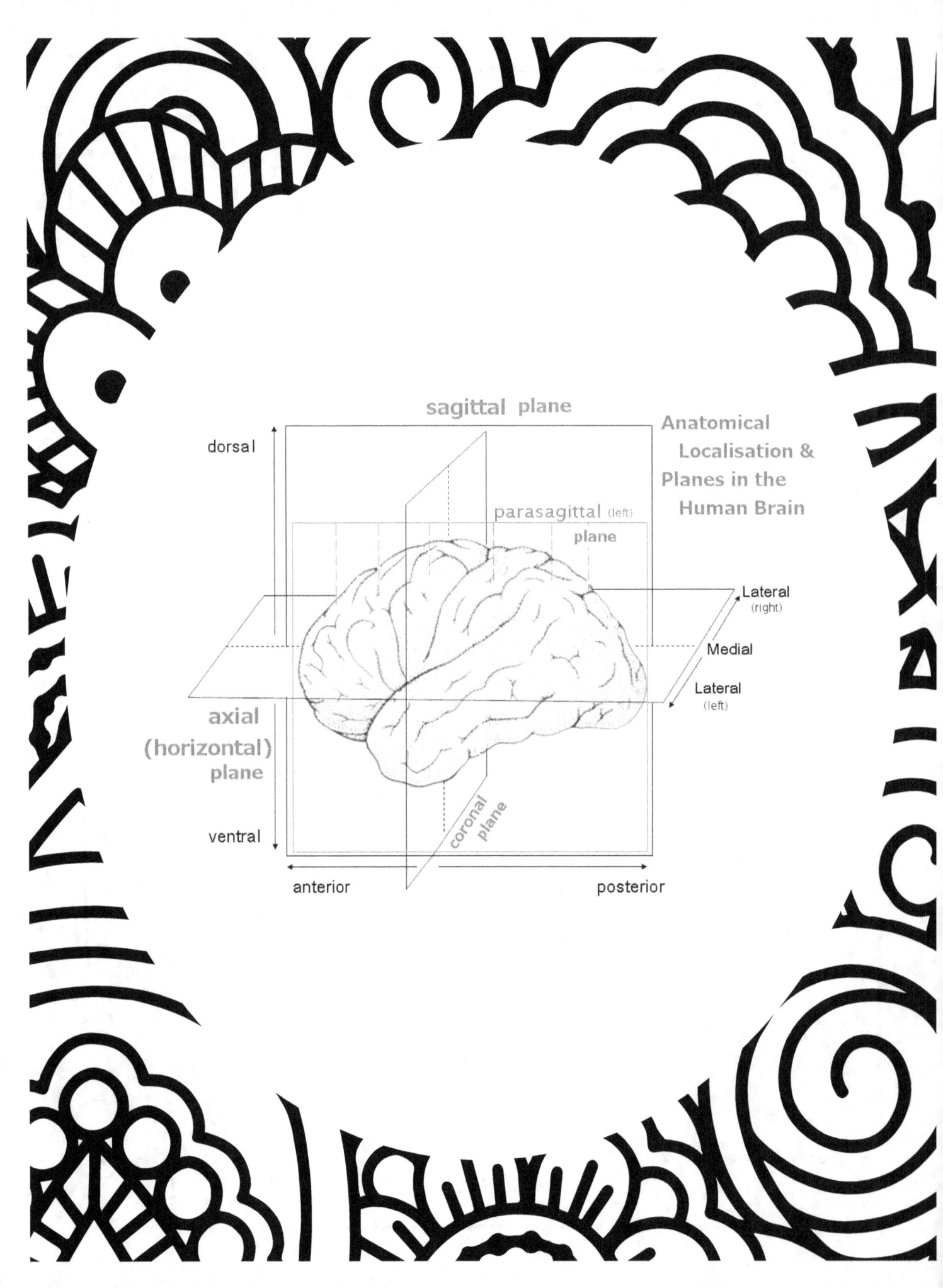

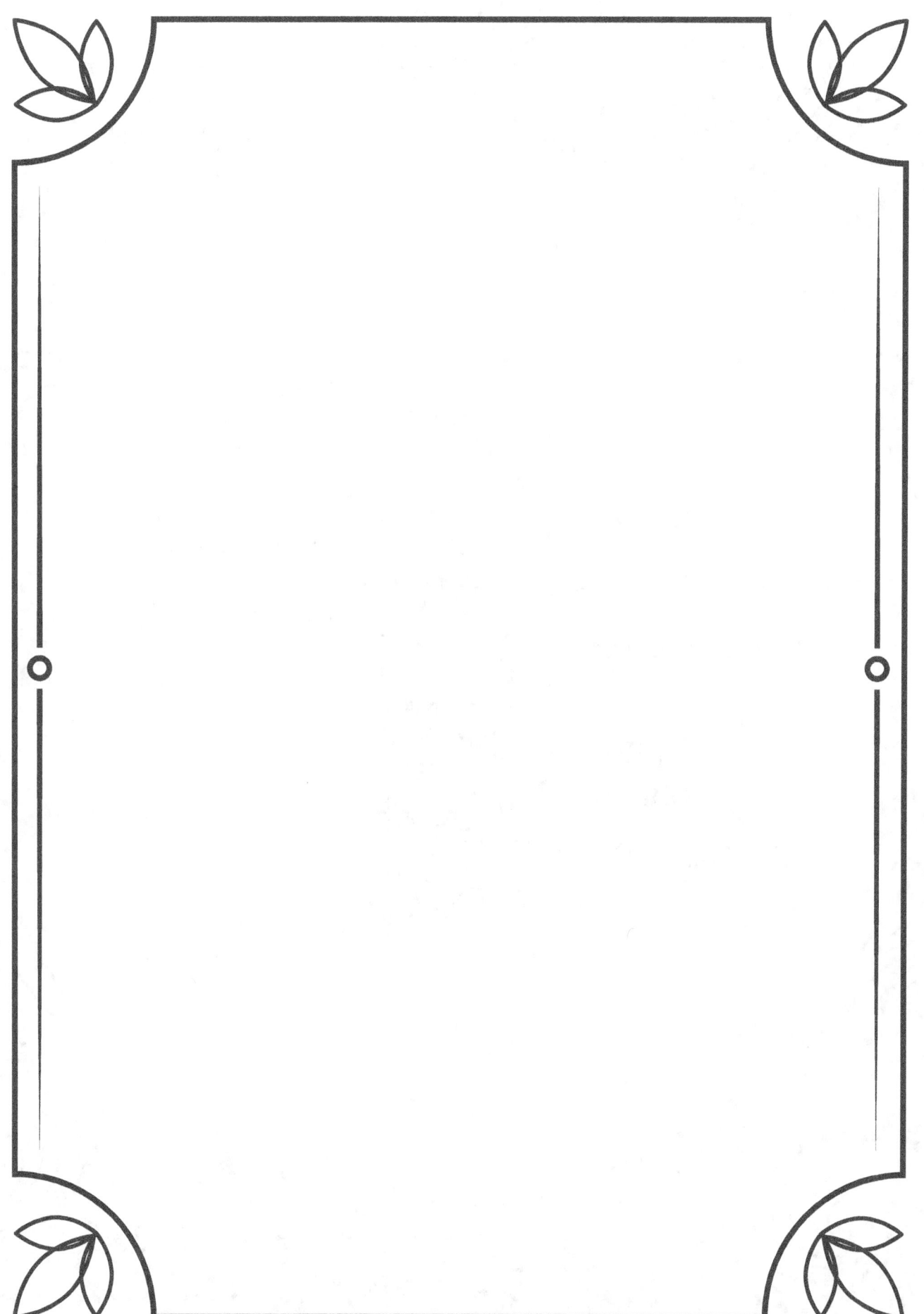

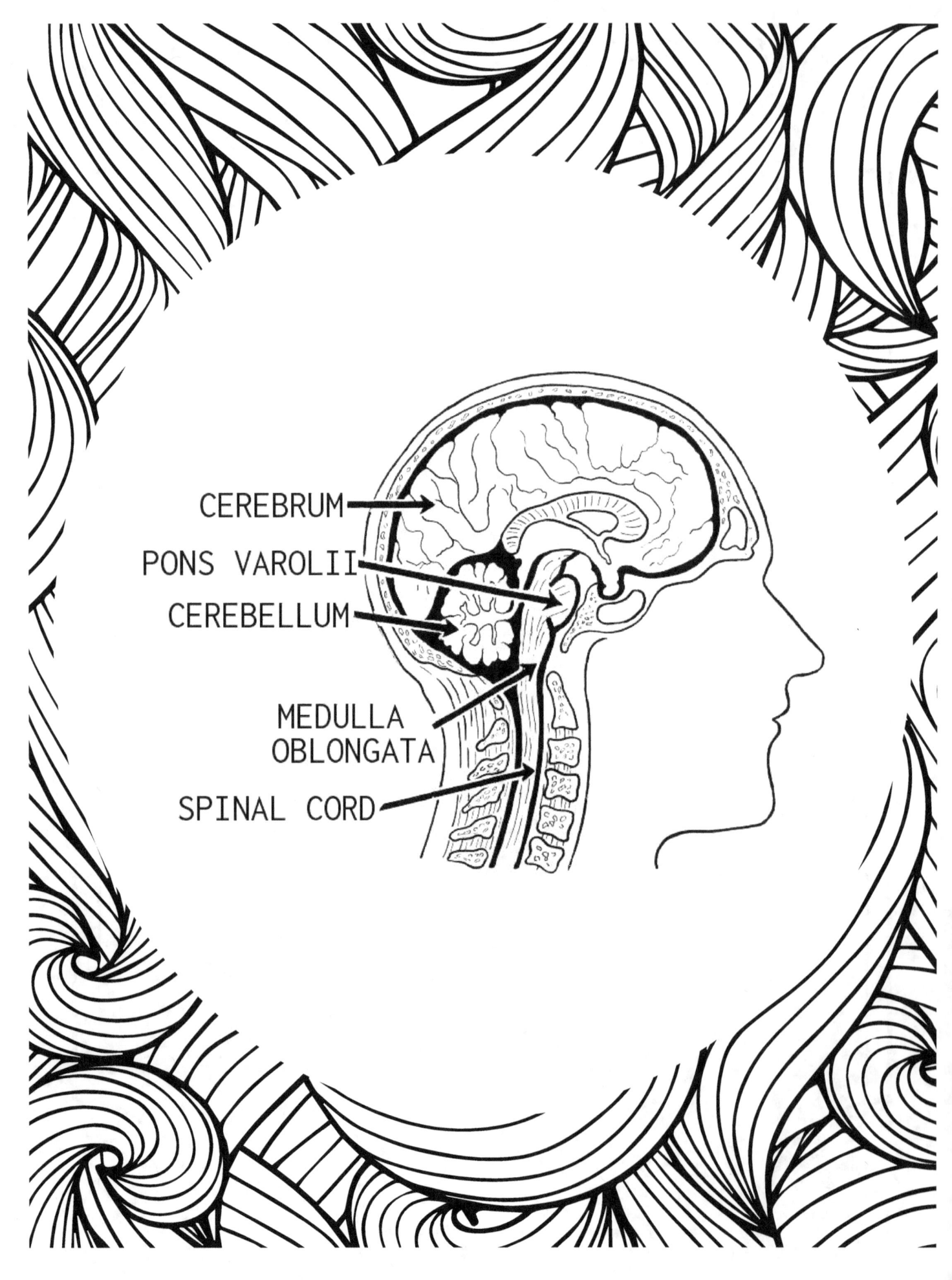

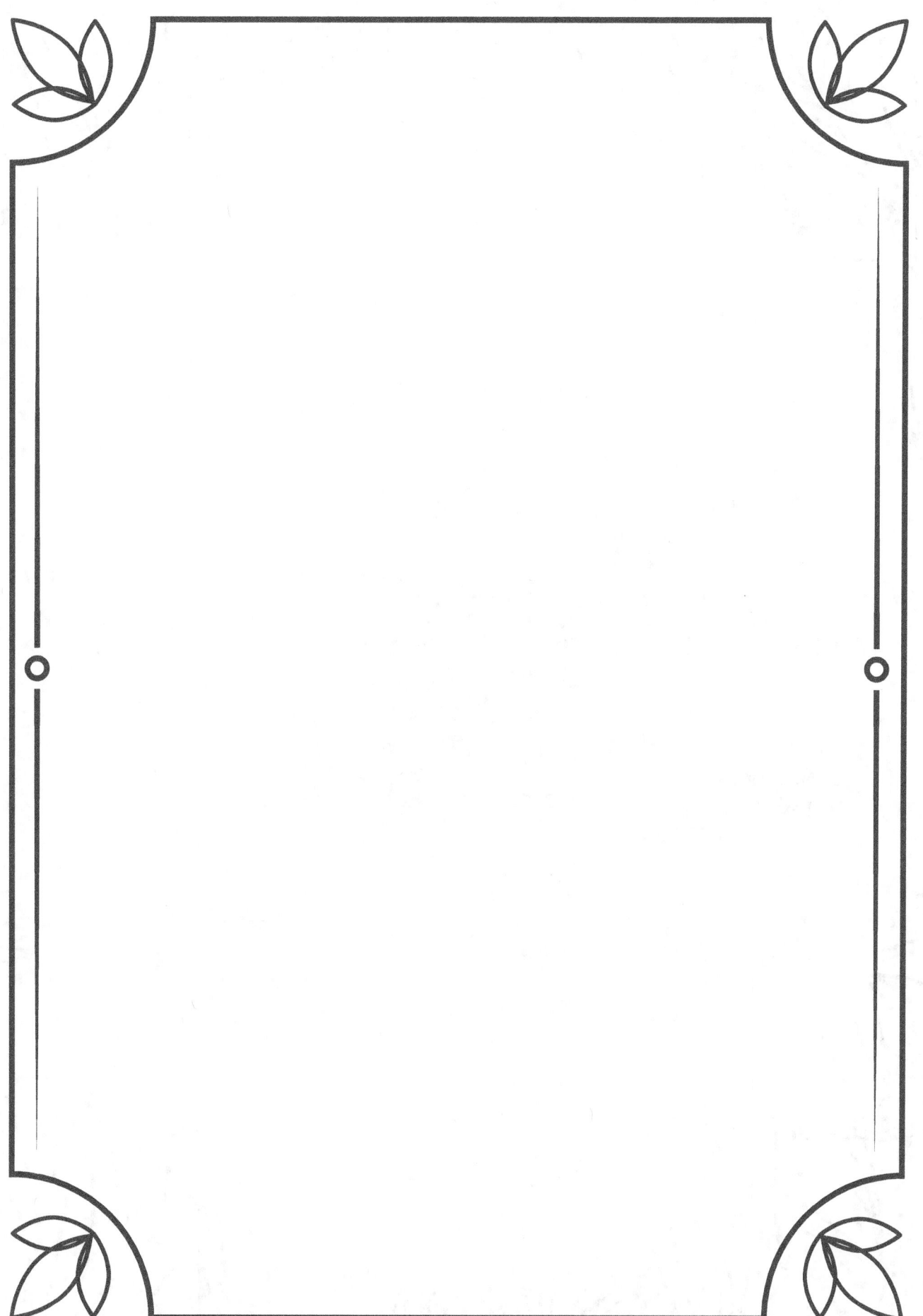

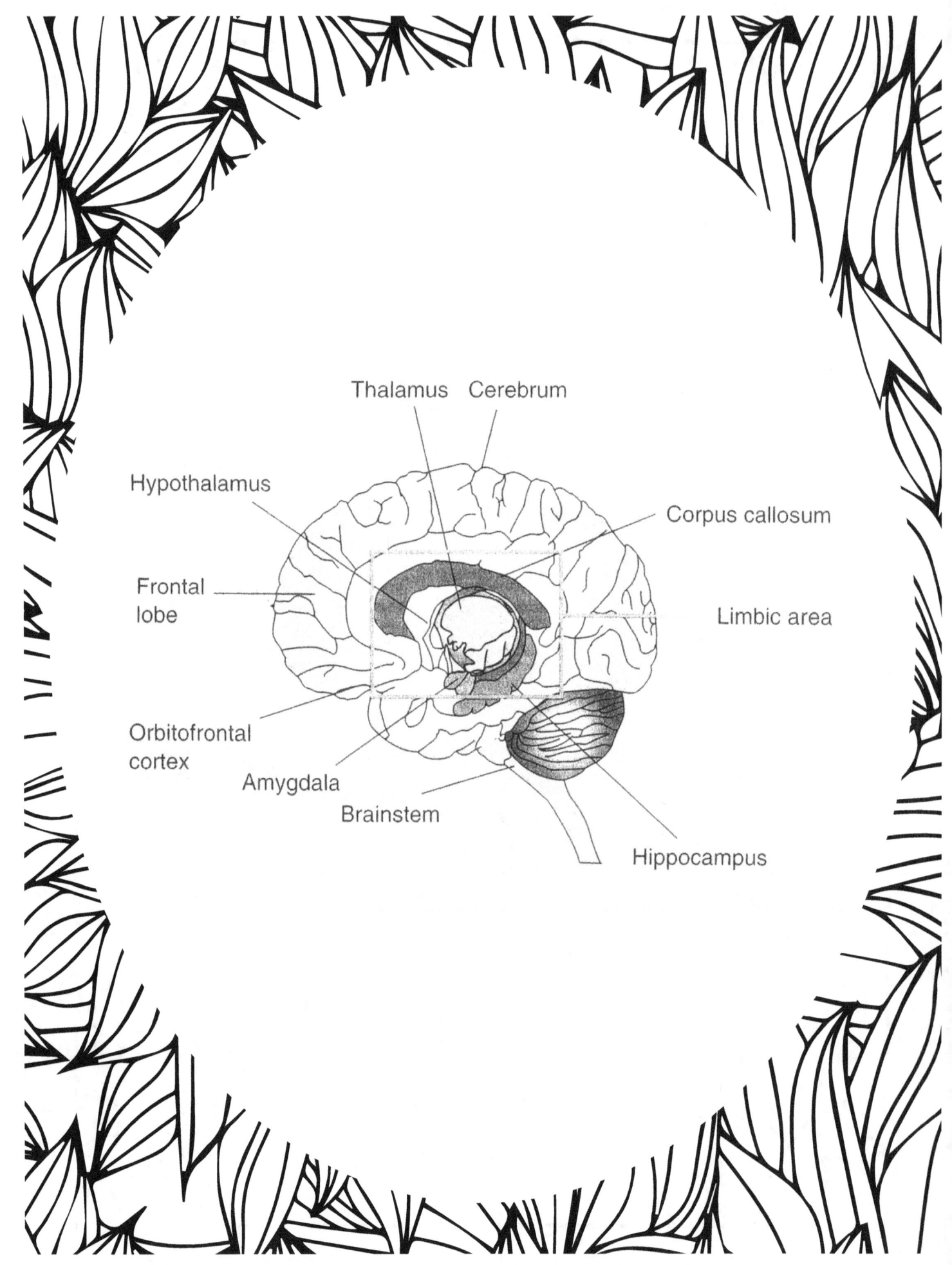

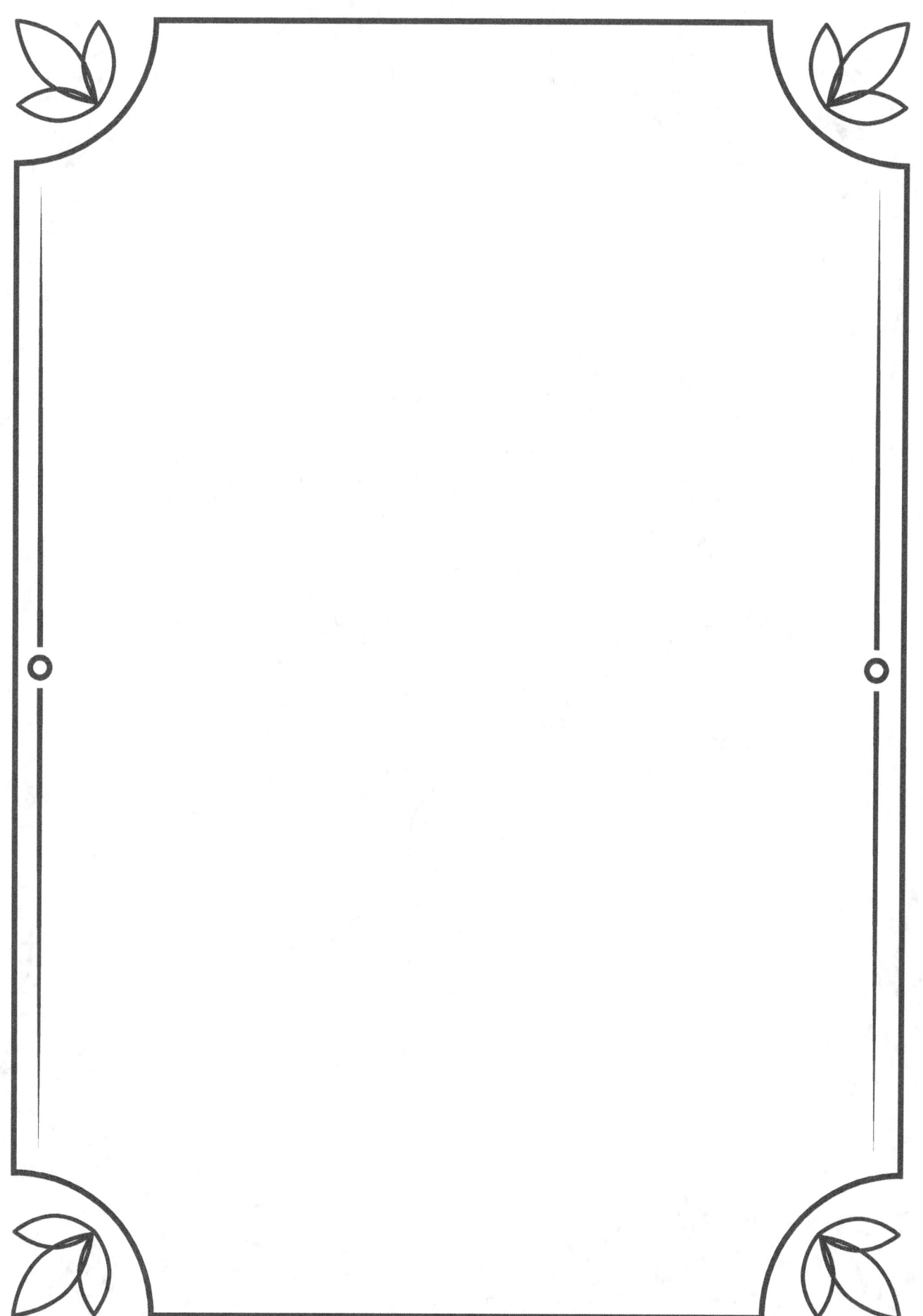

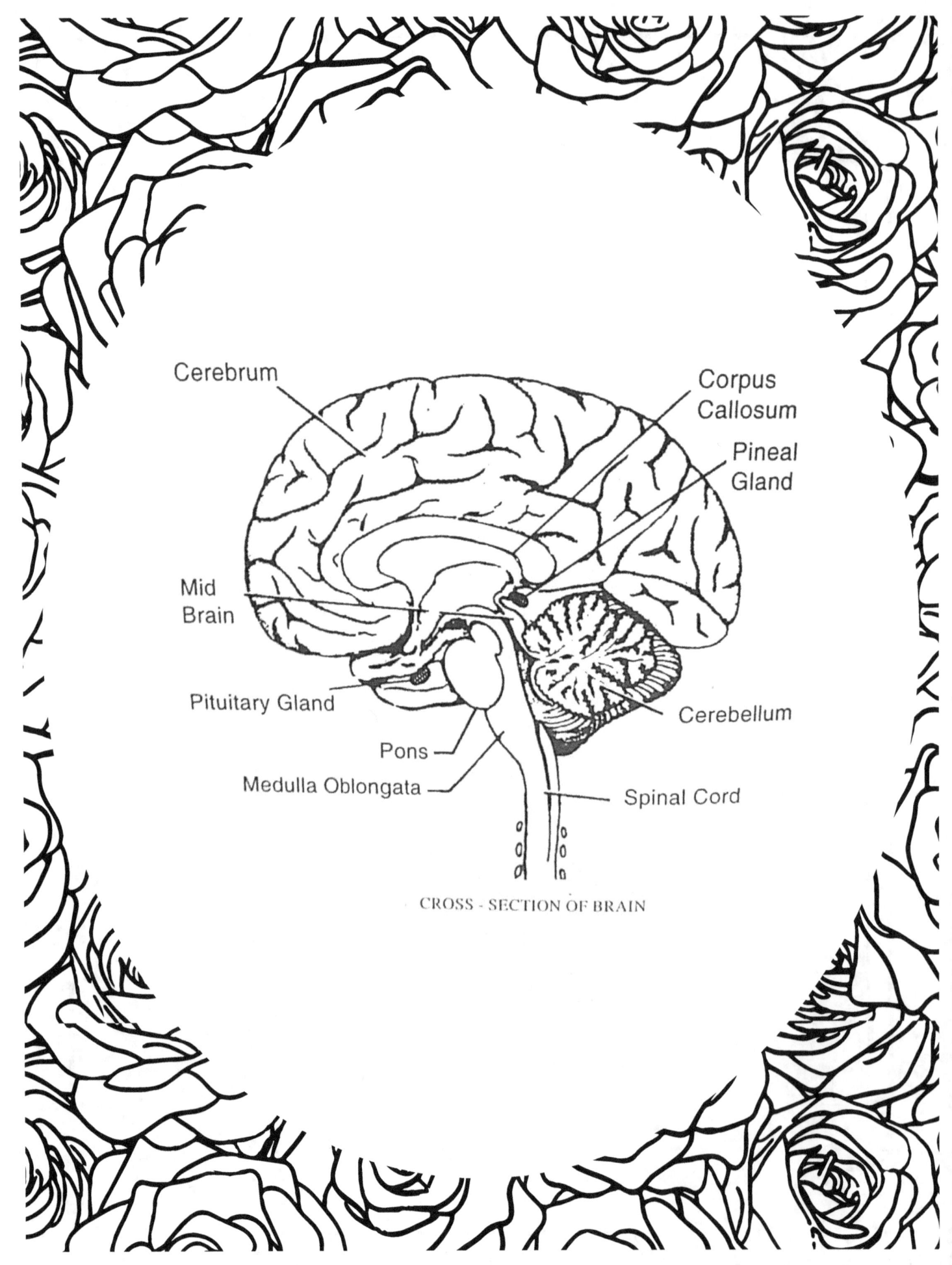

CROSS - SECTION OF BRAIN

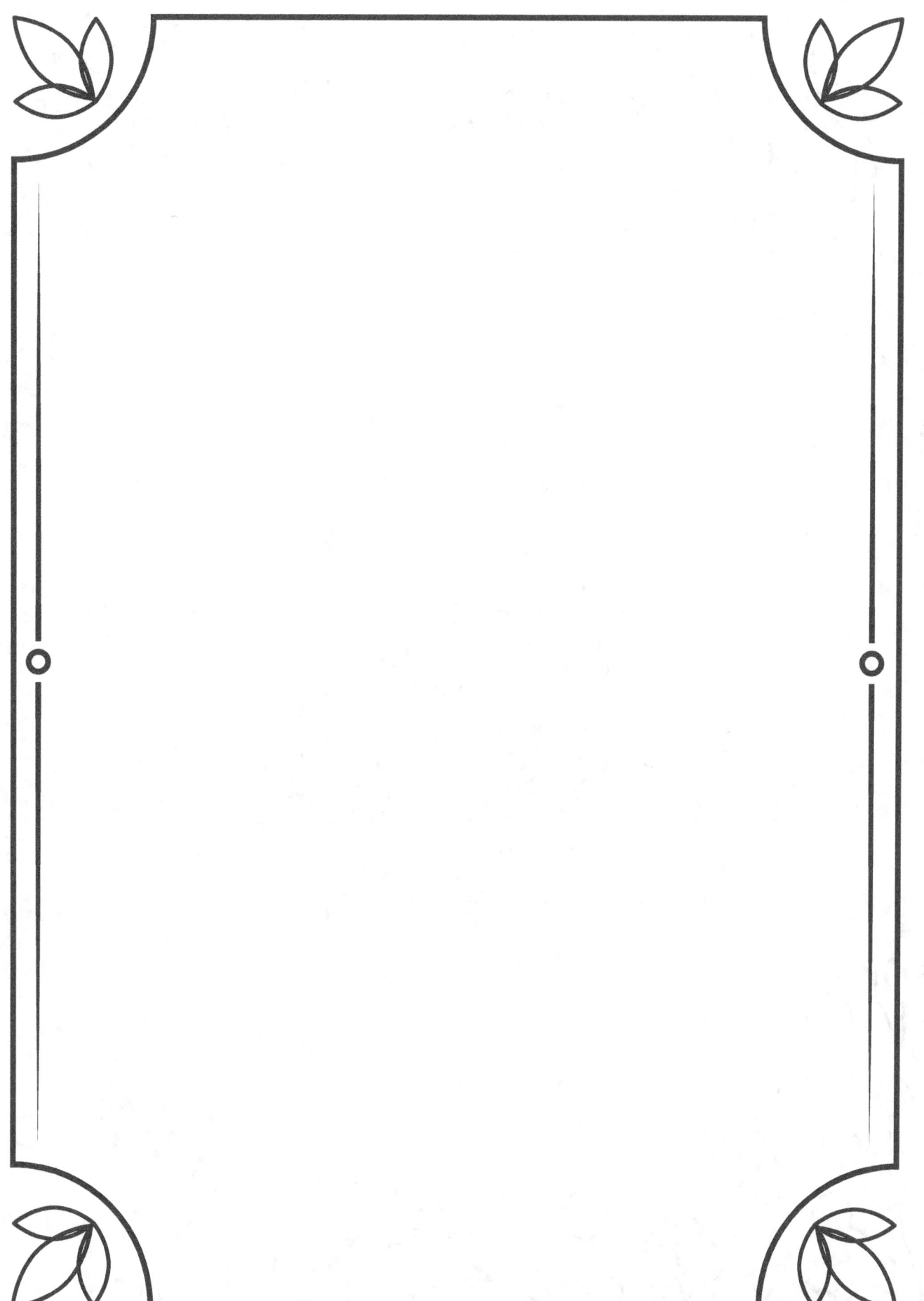

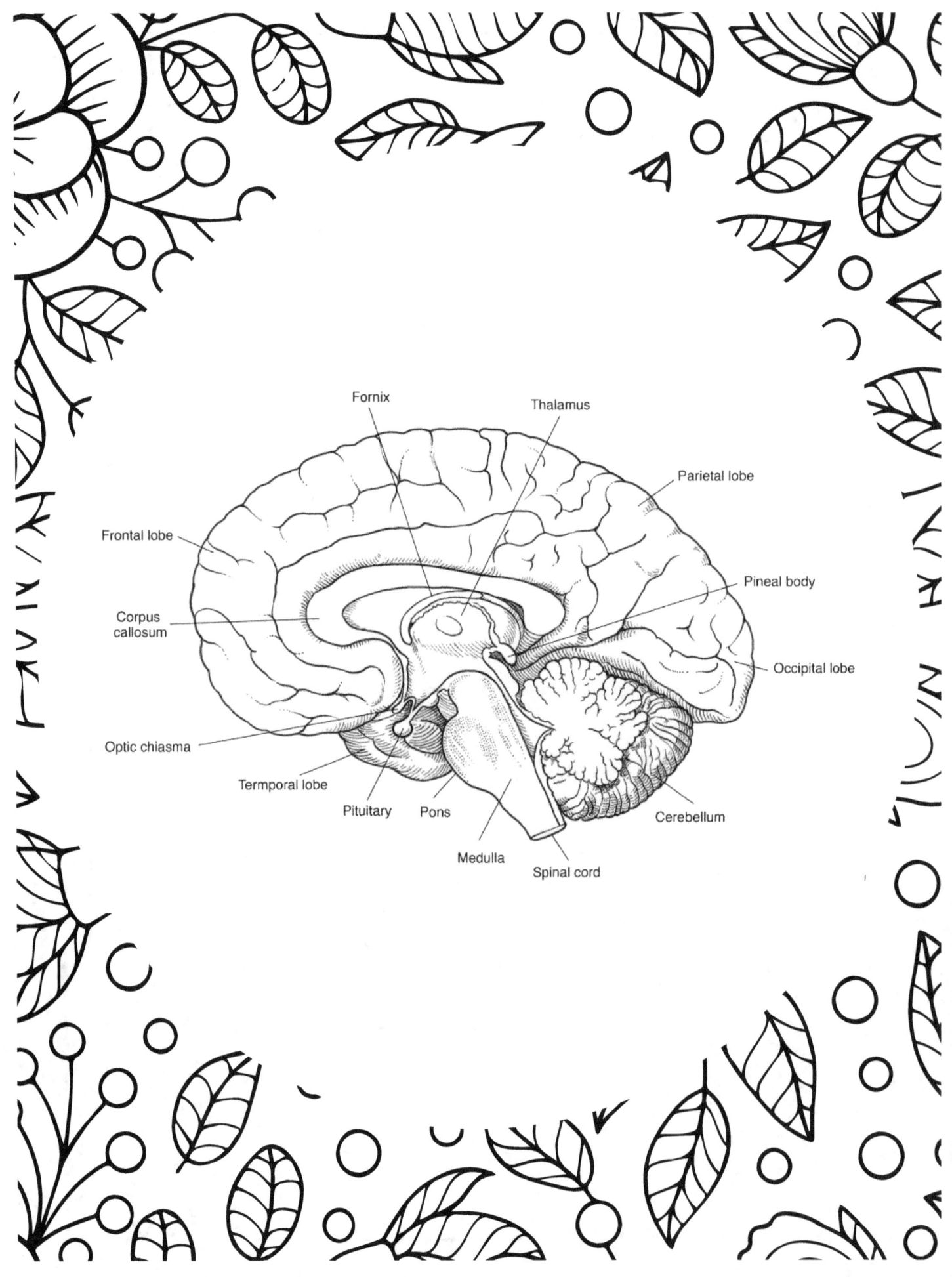

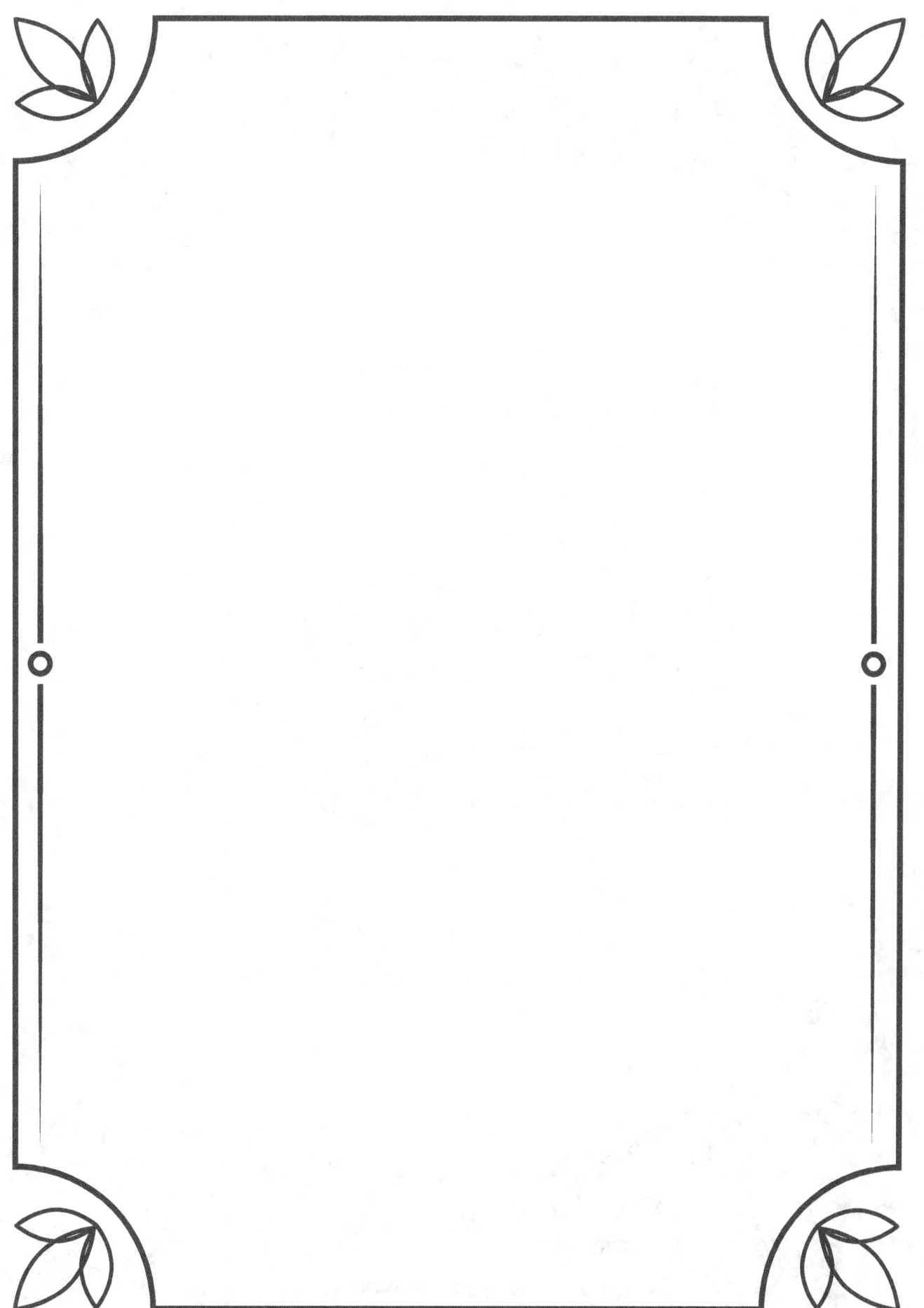

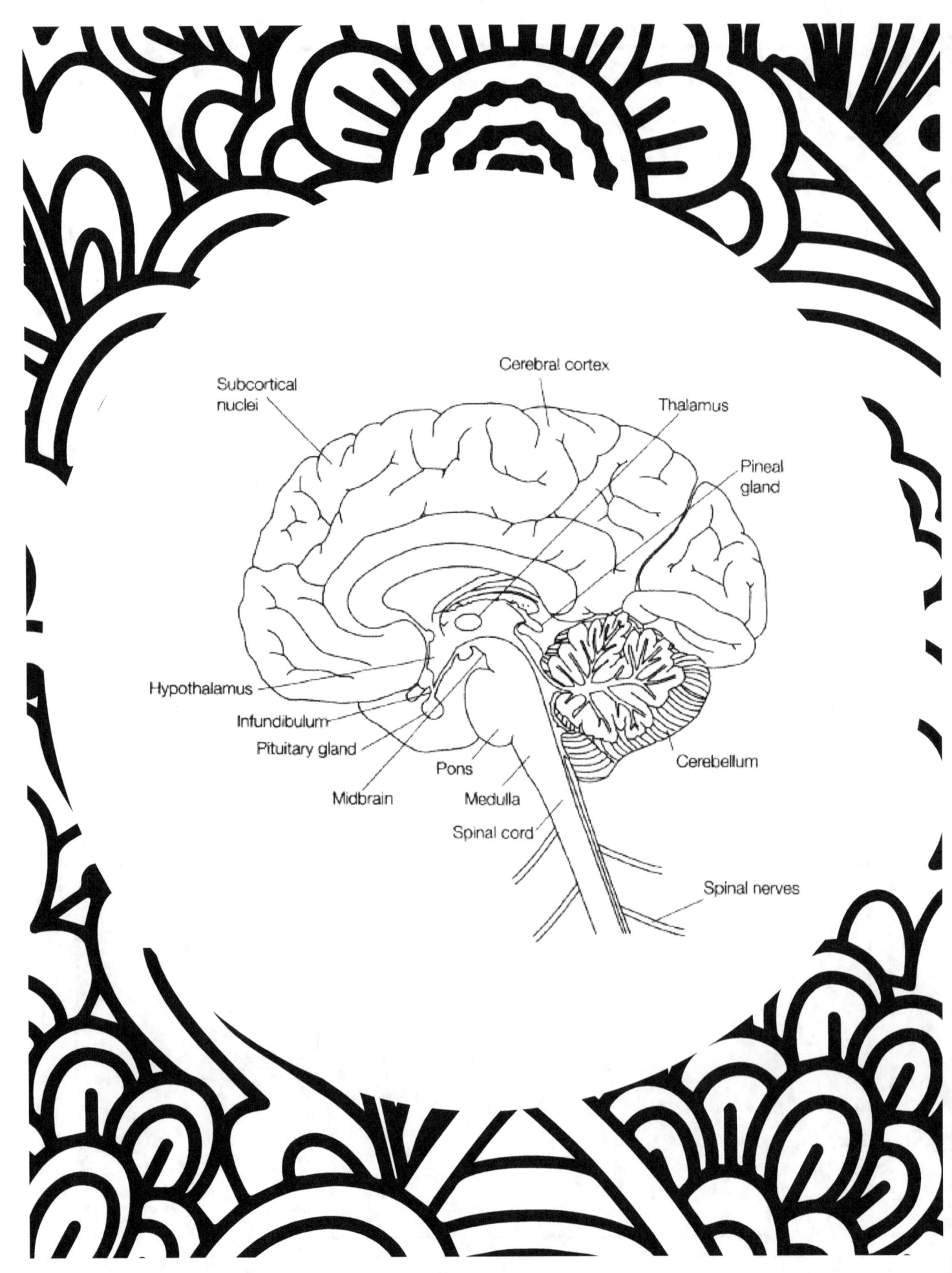

www.ingramcontent.com/pod-product-compliance
Lightning Source LLC
Chambersburg PA
CBHW081446220526
45466CB00008B/2527